O R L

OXFORD RHEUMATOLOGY LIBRARY

Axial Spondyloarthritis

O R L

OXFORD RHEUMATOLOGY LIBRARY

Axial Spondyloarthritis

Dr Stefan Siebert

Clinical Senior Lecturer in Rheumatology,
Institute of Infection, Immunity and Inflammation,
University of Glasgow

Dr Raj Sengupta

Consultant Rheumatologist, Royal National Hospital
for Rheumatic Diseases, Upper Borough Walls, Bath

Dr Alexander Tsoukas

Assistant Professor, McGill University, Montreal

OXFORD
UNIVERSITY PRESS

OXFORD
UNIVERSITY PRESS

Great Clarendon Street, Oxford, OX2 6DP,
United Kingdom

Oxford University Press is a department of the University of Oxford.
It furthers the University's objective of excellence in research, scholarship,
and education by publishing worldwide. Oxford is a registered trade mark of
Oxford University Press in the UK and in certain other countries

First Edition published in 2016

Impression: 1

Published in the United States of America by Oxford University Press
198 Madison Avenue, New York, NY 10016, United States of America

British Library Cataloguing in Publication Data
Data available

Library of Congress Control Number: 2016949670

ISBN 978–0–19–875529–6

Printed in Great Britain by
Ashford Colour Press Ltd, Gosport, Hampshire

Preface

Ankylosing spondylitis (AS) is a chronic inflammatory arthritis affecting mainly the sacroiliac joints and spine, resulting in pain, stiffness and reduced movement. Over the past decade there have been major advances in many aspects of the disease, including a broadening of the disease description to axial spondyloarthritis (axSpA). While the many advances have transformed the lives of patients with axSpA, they have also increased complexity for non-specialists in this area. Furthermore, many patients still present to a variety of healthcare professionals in primary and secondary care as first presentation, as part of their disease management or for an extra-articular manifestation or complication of their disease.

This handbook contains a timely update of the key developments and current state of play in axSpA for the many healthcare professionals who encounter patients with this condition, in both primary and secondary care settings. It will also be of interest to the wider medical and research community.

The handbook is written by rheumatologists with active research programmes and clinical expertise in these conditions. The topics covered herein include:

- the clinical features,
- extra-articular manifestations and complications,
- the impact on patients' lives,
- the major advances in genetics and pathogenesis,
- imaging advances (particularly MRI),
- classification criteria and diagnosis (and the important differences between these),
- non-pharmacological and drug treatments (with particular focus on TNF inhibitors and upcoming biologics) of axSpA.

This handbook will allow healthcare professionals who are not specialists in axSpA but who will encounter people with this condition in their clinical practice to ensure they are up-to-date with the many developments in this area and thereby ensure they are well placed to contribute to the optimal management and care for these patients.

Contents

List of Abbreviations

AAU	acute anterior uveitis
ACR	American College of Rheumatology
AP	antero-posterior
AS	ankylosing spondylitis
AS-WIS	Ankylosing Spondylitis Work Instability Scale
ASAS	Assessment of SpondyloArthritis international Society
ASAS20	ASAS 20% response
ASAS40	ASAS 40% response
ASDAS	Ankylosing Spondylitis Disease Activity Score
ASQoL	Ankylosing Spondylitis Quality of Life
axSpA	axial spondyloarthritis
BASDAI	Bath Ankylosing Spondyloarthritis Disease Activity Index
BASFI	Bath Ankylosing Spondylitis Functional Index
BAS-G	Bath Ankylosing Spondylitis Global
BASMI	Bath Ankylosing Spondylitis Metrology Index
BASRI	Bath Ankylosing Spondylitis Radiology Index
BMD	bone mineral density
BME	bone marrow oedema
CASPAR	ClASsification criteria for Psoriatic ARthritis
COX2	cyclo-oxygenase-2
CRP	C-reactive protein
CT	computed tomography
DAS28	28 joint disease activity score
DC-ART	disease-controlling anti-rheumatic treatment
DEXA	dual energy x-ray absorptiometry
DFI	Dougados Functional Index
DISH	diffuse idiopathic skeletal hyperostosis
DMARD	disease modifying anti-rheumatic drugs
EAM	extra-articular manifestation
EASi-QoL	Evaluation of Ankylosing Spondylitis quality of life
EMA	European Medicines Agency
ERAP	endoplasmic reticulum aminopeptidase

ESSG	European Spondylarthropathy Study Group
ESR	erythrocyte sedimentation rate
EULAR	European League Against Rheumatism
FDA	USA Food and Drug Administration
GWAS	genome-wide association studies
IBD	inflammatory bowel disease
IBP	inflammatory back pain
IL	interleukin
JAK	janus kinase
JIA	juvenile idiopathic arthritis
JSN	joint space narrowing
MASES	Maastricht Ankylosing Spondylitis Enthesitis Score
MCID	minimal clinically important difference
MHC	major histocompatibility complex
mNY	modified New York
MRI	magnetic resonance imaging
mSASSS	Modified Stoke Ankylosing Spondylitis Spine Score
NICE	National Institute for Health and Care Excellence
NSAID	non-steroidal anti-inflammatory drug
nr-axSpA	non-radiographic axSpA
NRS	numerical rating scale
PET	positron emission tomography
PGA	Patient Global Assessment
PRN	*pro re nata*
RA	rheumatoid arthritis
RA-WIS	Work Instability Scale for Rheumatoid Arthritis
RCT	randomized controlled trial
sDMARD	synthetic DMARDs
SI joints	sacroiliac joints
SM-ARDs	symptom modifying anti-rheumatic drugs
SpA	spondyloarthritis
SPARCC	Spondyloarthritis Research Consortium of Canada
STIR	short tau inversion recovery
TMJ	temporomandibular joint
TNF	tumour necrosis factor

VAS	visual analogue scale
WIS-RA	Work Instability Scale for Rheumatoid Arthritis
WLS	Work Limitations Questionnaire
WPAI:SpA	Work Productivity and Activity Impairment questionnaire in AS
WPS	Work Productivity Survey

Chapter 1

What are axial spondyloarthritis and ankylosing spondylitis?

Key points

- Ankylosing spondylitis (AS) is a chronic inflammatory arthritis affecting mainly the sacroiliac joints and spine, resulting in pain, stiffness, and reduced movement.
- AS has a major negative impact on patients' quality of life.
- AS is part of a larger group of related spondyloarthritis (SpA) conditions and patients with AS often have extra-articular manifestations of these conditions.
- Over the past decade, there have been major advances in the understanding of the genetics and pathophysiology of the disease.

Ankylosing spondylitis (AS) is a chronic inflammatory arthritis affecting mainly the sacroiliac joints and spine, resulting in pain, stiffness, and reduced movement. A diagnosis of AS requires a pre-defined level of radiographic (x-ray) damage of the sacroiliac joints and, in a significant number of patients, AS results in ankylosis (fusion) of the spine.

AS is associated with a range of related conditions, which include psoriasis, inflammatory bowel disease (IBD), and uveitis. These conditions share clinical, radiographic, and genetic factors, and have been collectively called the spondyloarthritides or spondyloarthritis (SpA). When features of these other conditions are present in a patient with AS, they are called extra-articular manifestations (EAMs) of AS. In addition to the spinal involvement and EAMs, AS can also be associated with peripheral musculoskeletal features, systemic fatigue, and an increased risk of certain complications.

The requirement for evidence of radiographic damage in order to make a diagnosis of AS led to long delays (average 10 years) from symptom onset to diagnosis. Furthermore, it was apparent that many patients had symptoms and disability consistent with AS but never developed the required degree of radiographic damage. These issues became particularly pressing with the development of TNF inhibitors for the treatment of AS. In parallel, advances in magnetic resonance imaging (MRI) enabled the detection of inflammatory changes of sacroiliac joints and the spine prior to the development of structural radiographic damage. As a result, the Assessment of SpondyloArthritis international Society (ASAS) developed validated classification criteria for axial spondyloarthritis (axSpA). These criteria allowed a patient with chronic back pain to be classified with axSpA via imaging or clinical (but no imaging) routes. Furthermore, the imaging arm included the option of either MRI evidence of inflammatory sacroiliitis or radiographic x-ray evidence of structural damage. Imaging of the spine is not yet included in the current classification criteria. While these classification criteria were developed for use in research studies, they have facilitated the earlier diagnosis and treatment of patients with axSpA in clinical practice.

However, the issue of diagnosis and nomenclature remain complex and often misunderstood in this area. The classification criteria cannot simply be applied to patients presenting to clinicians in daily practice, although this appears to be relatively common practice. Diagnosis still requires careful assessment by a specialist with expertise in axSpA, taking into account context, pre-test probability, and potential alternative diagnoses. The current view is that AS and axSpA are part of the same spectrum, and there is increasingly a move towards using axSpA as the main diagnostic term. The term 'AS' would then indicate a patient with axSpA who has evidence of radiographic damage on x-ray of the sacroiliac joints, while the term 'non-radiographic' axSpA (nr-axSpA) refers to a patient with axSpA but no radiographic changes.

While issues remain to be resolved, there have undoubtedly been major advances in AS and axSpA over the past decade. AS has essentially gone from a condition that was only diagnosed late, once structural damage was already present, with very limited treatment options, to a condition that can now be diagnosed increasingly early and treated with highly effective biologic agents for those with severe disease. There have also been major advances in the understanding of the genetics and pathophysiology of the condition, which has led to the development of new therapeutic agents for SpA which should be available in the clinic for axSpA in the next few years. These changes have combined to transform the lives of patients with axSpA.

Historical perspective

Evidence of skeletal changes consistent with AS have been reported for several centuries, with the clinical features described in the late 19th century. The development of radiology further facilitated the diagnosis. In the early 1900s, it was increasingly recognized that AS was distinct from rheumatoid arthritis (RA) and was instead associated with a number of other conditions such as psoriasis, IBD, and uveitis. This led to the concept of SpA, with shared clinical, radiographic, and hereditary features. The discovery of the strong association with HLA-B27 and then the more recent advances in imaging, immunopathogenesis, genetics, and treatment have transformed the lives of these patients, particularly compared to their predecessors in earlier centuries. Historical perspectives are covered in more detail in Chapter 2.

Epidemiological perspective

Chronic low back pain remains a leading cause of disability worldwide. A small, but significant proportion of these patients will have inflammatory back pain (IBP), of which a further proportion will have axSpA or another SpA-related condition. There is a paucity of good epidemiological studies to define the true incidence and prevalence of AS, axSpA, and SpA, with wide variation as a result of geographic, demographic, and methodological factors. Furthermore, there is also significant heterogeneity in the natural history and progression of axSpA. Epidemiological perspectives are covered in more detail in Chapter 3.

Genetic, immunologic, and pathophysiological perspectives

Family and twin studies have long suggested a large genetic component in AS, which was confirmed by the discovery of the strong association with HLA-B27. The exact mechanism by which HLA-B27 contributes to AS remains unknown, with three main theories proposed: the arthritogenic peptide, endoplasmic reticulum stress with unfolded protein response, and homodimerization theories. More recently, genome-wide association studies have identified a number of other important susceptibility genes, most notably ERAP1 and IL-23R. Genetic, immunologic and pathophysiological perspectives are covered in more detail in Chapters 4 and 5.

While the exact pathophysiology of axSpA remains unclear, significant advances have recently been made and suggest a potential role and interplay of genetic susceptibility, biomechanics, the microbiome, and key cytokine pathways. The IL-23/IL-17 cytokine pathway, in particular, has been increasingly implicated and is leading to the development of potential new therapies for axSpA.

Axial and peripheral musculoskeletal manifestations

Chronic back pain is the commonest presenting feature in axSpA, but only a small fraction of people with this very common symptom will have axSpA. However, there are some symptoms that may help distinguish IBP from the far more prevalent non-specific or mechanical back pain. Therefore, recognizing the features of IBP is often an important first step in identifying potential patients with axSpA and a number of validated criteria for IBP have been proposed. However, IBP does not equate to a diagnosis of axSpA and many patients with IBP will not have axSpA.

In addition to the axial involvement which characterizes axSpA, a proportion of patients also develop peripheral musculoskeletal involvement. This can include synovitis of joints, enthesitis, and dactylitis. Many of these features may be relatively subtle, although they can have a significant impact on patient outcomes and quality of life. In particular, hip involvement is a bad prognostic feature which often warrants more aggressive therapy. Axial and peripheral musculoskeletal manifestations are covered in more detail in Chapters 6 and 7.

Extra-articular manifestations and complications of axSpA

In addition to the well-recognized inflammatory musculoskeletal manifestations, axSpA is also associated with a number of other features. These EAMs reflect shared clinical, genetic, and pathophysiological features with the other SpA-related conditions. The key EAMs of axSpA are uveitis, IBD, and psoriasis. The EAMs carry their own morbidity and often warrant treatment in their own right. The identification, monitoring, and treatment of EAMs is an important part of the management of patients with axSpA.

While the EAMs are considered part of the SpA spectrum, patients may also develop a range of complications as a consequence of having the disease. Patients with AS are at increased risk of osteoporosis and spinal fractures. The latter may occur after seemingly minor trauma and may lead to significant neurological compromise. Patients may also develop other neurological complications, including atlantoaxial subluxation, compressive radiculopathy or myelopathy. Cardiac complications include cardiovascular events, increased hypertension, valvular disease and conduction disturbances. Pulmonary disease in AS relates to parenchymal involvement or mechanical constraint from chest wall inflammation, while renal disease is generally rare in AS. The EAMs and complications of axSpA are covered in more detail in Chapters 8 and 9.

The impact and cost of axSpA

Patients with axSpA consistently report lower health-related quality of life compared to the general population, with a similar burden of disease reported for nr-axSpA and established AS. The effects of the condition include factors such as pain, reduced mobility, poor sleep, fatigue, and depression. AxSpA also significantly impacts on social and work participation, with lower work participation and higher early retirement rates. Those patients in work also report reduced work productivity due to absenteeism (ability to attend work) and presenteeism (productivity while at work). While estimates of the total cost of AS vary greatly, particularly between countries, studies consistently indicate that the majority of the costs associated with AS are due to work-related factors. The impact and cost of axSpA are covered in more detail in Chapter 10.

Imaging in axSpA

Imaging has always been a key component in the diagnosis of AS. With the increased availability of MRI and the development of the ASAS axSpA criteria, there has been a shift from x-ray imaging of structural damage to MRI imaging of active inflammation. This information can help in both the diagnosis of axSpA and in guiding treatment decisions in these patients. Advances in technology are likely to lead to the development of even better imaging modalities for axSpA in future. Imaging in axSpA is covered in more detail in Chapter 11.

Classification criteria and diagnosis

There is no single 'gold standard' clinical, laboratory, pathologic, or radiologic feature to confirm the diagnosis of axSpA. A number of criteria for AS and axSpA have, therefore, been developed to support clinical practice and research. The ASAS criteria for axSpA are currently the most widely used classification criteria, although it is likely that these will continue to evolve in future as understanding of SpA advances. The ASAS axSpA criteria can be fulfilled by a number of routes and allow patients to be classified as nr-axSpA (fulfill pre-defined MRI or clinical features) or AS (fulfill radiographic x-ray features), although these are considered to be part of the same spectrum of disease (namely axSpA) rather than separate diseases. Significantly, the ASAS axSpA criteria have allowed biologic therapies to be investigated, and used, in earlier disease and for a wider population of patients.

However, these are classification criteria developed for use in research studies and cannot therefore simply be applied for diagnostic purposes in routine clinical practice. There remains significant misunderstanding about the important differences between classification and diagnostic criteria. Diagnosis still requires careful assessment by a physician, ideally a specialist with expertise in axSpA, taking into account context, pre-test probability, and potential alternative diagnoses, rather than a checklist approach using classification criteria. Classification criteria and diagnosis is covered in more detail in Chapter 12.

Assessment and monitoring outcomes

Monitoring outcomes has become an increasingly important aspect in the management of axSpA, with a number of assessments mandatory in those patients receiving biologic therapies. There are an increasingly large number of potential outcomes that can be assessed, including patient-reported and clinician-assessed measures assessing disease activity, symptoms (such as pain, stiffness and fatigue), function, mobility, work disability, and quality of life. In selected patients, acute phase blood tests and imaging may also play a role in the monitoring axSpA, and it is likely that in future there will be an increasing move towards more objective measures. Assessment and monitoring outcomes are covered in more detail in Chapter 13.

Treatment perspectives

Even in the era of biologic drugs, the optimal management of axSpA requires a combination of non-pharmacological and pharmacological treatments, for both initial and long-term management. Non-drug therapies are crucial in maintaining function, mobility, and quality of life. Regular physical therapy and exercise remain mainstays of non-drug management, combined with self-management and education strategies. A proportion of patients with severe disease may also require hip or spinal surgery.

Until approximately 2005, treatment options were limited to exercise therapy and non-steroidal anti-inflammatory drugs (NSAIDs). The management of patients with axSpA, especially those with severe disease, has been transformed by the introduction of anti-TNF therapy. The TNF inhibitors appear to have a good safety profile in axSpA, with no new safety signals. The high cost of innovator biologics remains an issue, and it will be interesting to observe the effect of the introduction of multiple biosimilar TNF inhibitors in clinical practice. Newer therapeutics targeting different cytokine and signalling pathways, particularly the IL-23/IL-17 axis, should also become available over the next few years, so it remains to be seen what their role will be in the management of axSpA. Treatment perspectives are covered in more detail in Chapters 14 and 15.

Chapter 2

A brief history of ankylosing spondylitis

Key points

- The history of ankylosing spondylitis (AS) dates back to the discovery of 5000-year-old skeletons with characteristic spinal changes.
- Numerous cases of AS have featured in medical literature since the 16th century.
- The disease was further defined by correlating pathological and clinical features, and the development of clinical radiology.
- Subsequent epidemiological and familial studies highlighted the association with other conditions as part of the spondyloarthritides. The discovery of HLA-B27 confirmed this association.
- Over the past two decades, genome-wide association studies, and advances in imaging and immunology have yielded dramatic insights into the disease and the development of highly effective therapies.

The earliest evidence of ankylosing spondylitis (AS) may date back to ancient Egypt, where paleopathological analysis of the skeletons of 5000-year-old mummified pharaohs showed spinal osteophyte formation and 'bamboo spines' suggestive of the disease. However, this still remains controversial as definitive distinction from diffuse idiopathic skeletal hyperostosis (DISH) is difficult.

The first published cases in medical literature were in 1559 when Realdo Colombo, an assistant to Andreas Vesalius at the University of Padua, described two skeletons with spinal disease suggestive of AS. In his excellent review, Bywaters called this the 'fossil stage' in the development of the history of AS (Bywaters, 1979). Several other pathological descriptions of medieval skeletons described changes typical of AS, but, the first definite description of AS is attributed to Bernard Connor (1666–1695), an

Irish physician studying at the University of Rheims. While demonstrating anatomy, he noted a male skeleton in which complete bone fusion had occurred from the lower ribcage and thoracic spine to the sacrum. In his thesis (1691), he postulated the man probably had difficulty breathing due to fused rib joints, and trouble turning and bending due to the spinal fusion. In the mid-1800s, several clinical cases were described in Europe for the first time, with clinical and post-mortem pathology correlation suggesting links between the spinal and extra-spinal manifestations (including iritis) in the patients.

In 1893, Vladimir von Bekhterev, a Russian neurologist and psychologist, described a series of three patients, including a mother and daughter, who had previous back trauma and developed a form of *spondylitis deformans*. He postulated that a chronic inflammatory process of the vertebrae had led to rigidity, bone fusion, and myelopathy, and that it had a hereditary component. Adolph Strümpell (1897) and Pierre Marie (1898), neurologists from Germany and France, respectively, characterized further cases and independently delineated the disease as being primarily rheumatological. These descriptions, together with the development of radiology in the late 1800s, facilitated the ability to diagnose the disease prior to the development of severe ankylosis. For these reasons, AS was previously also known as Bechterew's Disease (the transliteration of Bekhterev) or Marie-Strümpell Disease, terms which are still used in some countries.

The x-ray changes of AS were characterized in the early 1900s by Forestier, Scott, Krebs and others who described sacroiliac joint arthritis early in the disease, with later syndesmophyte formation. The disease appeared to be familial and epidemiological studies were carried out to investigate inheritance patterns. However, many rheumatologists at the time believed this disease to be a clinical subset of rheumatoid arthritis (RA) affecting the spine, which was occasionally triggered by factors such as psoriasis, colitis, and urethritis. While many 'lumped' AS as a subset of RA, the striking difference in x-ray findings and lack of rheumatoid factor prompted others to 'split' it into a completely different disease category of seronegative arthritis.

From the 1930s until the mid-1950s radiation therapy was widely used for the treatment of AS. While this was often very effective, it was subsequently abandoned due to the concern about secondary malignancies as a result of this treatment. A follow-up study in the United Kingdom of 14,000 patients with AS who had received at least one x-ray course revealed a threefold increase in mortality for leukaemia and a 28% increase in mortality from neoplasms other than leukaemia or colon cancer, compared to the general population.

By the 1950s, not only was the distinction with RA indisputable, but association with the other seronegative arthritides was increasingly recognized.

Marche (1954) and Oates (1959) (both cited in Zeidler, 2011) suggested that AS and Reiter's syndrome (now called reactive arthritis) were associated and may share the same origin, while Amor (1968; also cited in cited in Zeidler, 2011) postulated a common genetic background after noting the frequent development of AS in those with Reiter's syndrome.

A year after Moll and Wright proposed their seminal classification for psoriatic arthritis, they also proposed a unifying concept for a group of related seronegative arthritides which included AS, psoriatic arthritis, Reiter's disease, intestinal arthropathies, and Behcet's syndrome. This group of conditions, termed spondyloarthritides, share common characteristics including negative rheumatoid factor, absence of 'rheumatoid' nodules, peripheral inflammatory arthritis, radiologic sacroiliitis, tendency to familial aggregation, and related clinical features such as psoriasis, uveitis, conjunctivitis, intestinal inflammation, and genitourinary infections.

While the familial tendency in AS had been recognized in the 19th century, and a genetic link between the various seronegative diseases was postulated, this remained unproven until the 1970s. In 1973, two groups independently described the HLA-B27 association with AS, representing one of the strongest genetic associations ever reported in a polygenic disease (see Chapter 4). Of interest, HLA-B27 sequences were subsequently detected in the skeletal remains of presumed AS cases from the Middle Ages. Subsequent studies also indicated the association of HLA-B27 with Reiter's syndrome and psoriatic arthritis, supporting the concept of spondyloarthritides as a family of diseases sharing similar pathogenetic manifestations. The concept of spondyloarthritis (SpA) was subsequently incorporated into disease classification criteria and remains important in clinical practice (covered in Chapter 12).

Following the discovery of the association with HLA-B27, progress in genetics largely stalled and the treatment of AS remained largely limited to physiotherapy and non-steroidal anti-inflammatory drugs throughout the late twentieth century (see Chapter 15). However, over the past two decades, large genome-wide association studies, advances in imaging, and increased understanding of immunology (see Chapters 4, 5, and 11) have led to novel insights into the disease processes and the development of both new classification criteria and therapies, transforming the lives of patients with this condition.

Key References and further reading:

Bywaters, EG. Historical aspects of ankylosing spondylitis. *Rheumatol Rehabil.* 1979;**18**(4):197–203. doi: 10.1093/rheumatology/18.4.197

Moll JM, Haslock I, Macrae IF, Wright V. Associations between ankylosing spondylitis, psoriatic arthritis, Reiter's disease, the intestinal arthropathies, and Behcet's syndrome. *Medicine.* 1974;**53**(5):343–64. PMID: 4604133

Sieper J, Braun J, Rudwaleit M, *et al.* Ankylosing spondylitis: an overview. *Ann Rheum Dis.* 2002;**61**(Suppl 3):iii8–18. doi: 10.1136/ard.61.suppl_3.iii8

Zeidler H, Calin A, Amor B. A historical perspective of the spondyloarthritis. *Curr Opin Rheumatol.* 2011;**23**(4):327–333. doi: 10.1097/BOR.0b013e3283470ecd

Chapter 3

The epidemiology of ankylosing spondylitis, axial spondyloarthritis, and back pain

Key points

- Low back pain is a leading cause of disability worldwide. The prevalence of inflammatory back pain (IBP) has been calculated to be in the range 8–15% in a UK primary care population and 5–7% in a USA population-based cohort.
- There is a paucity of good epidemiological studies to define the true incidence and prevalence of ankylosing spondylitis (AS), axial spondyloarthritis (axSpA), and spondyloarthritis (SpA), with wide variation as a result of geographic, demographic, and methodological factors.
- The global prevalence estimates are in the range 0.01–0.2% for AS, 0.32–0.7% for axSpA and around 1% for SpA overall.
- The global incidence estimates are in the range 0.44–7.3 cases per 100,000 person-years for AS and 0.48–62.5 cases per 100,000 person-years for SpA.

There is a paucity of good epidemiological studies to define the real incidence and prevalence of ankylosing spondylitis (AS) and axial spondyloarthritis (axSpA). Furthermore, most of the published epidemiological studies pre-date the development of the Assessment of SpondyloArthritis international Society (ASAS) criteria in 2009. Therefore, most of the data relates to AS rather than the broader axSpA spectrum. By definition, AS incorporates only patients who already have established radiographic changes, so reflects a later stage of the axSpA spectrum, although not all patients with non-radiographic axSpA (nr-axSpA) will go on to develop AS.

Chronic low back pain

Low back pain is a leading cause of disability worldwide and the second most common symptom-related reason for visiting a doctor in the USA. Approximately 60–80% of the UK population will experience back pain at some point in their lives. Interestingly, a lower mean lifetime prevalence of low back pain has been reported in low–middle income countries.

In the majority of patients, episodes of acute back pain will resolve, but a significant proportion will develop chronic back pain which is where the burden of disability and health-related costs resides. A recent systematic review reported a global prevalence of chronic low back pain (defined as pain lasting ≥3 months) ranging from 10.3% to 29.9%. There are many possible causes for chronic low back pain, with the majority due to mechanical and degenerative causes (see Box 6.1 for causes of chronic back pain). Studies have shown that up to 5% of patients with chronic back pain have AS, with the prevalence varying in line with the *HLA-B27* gene in a given population. In the UK, approximately 7% of the general population is HLA-B27 positive, while approximately 92% of patients with known AS are HLA-B27 positive. It should be noted, that the majority of people who are HLA-B27 positive do not have AS.

Inflammatory back pain (IBP) is the key presenting symptom in AS and axSpA (covered in more detail in Chapter 6). However, there is limited information about the true prevalence of IBP. In a cross-sectional cohort study, the prevalence of IBP in a UK primary care population with back pain was 8% using the ASAS criteria and 13–15% using the older Calin and Berlin criteria (see Chapter 6 for more information on the IBP criteria). There was no significant difference between men and women. The prevalence of IBP in a large US population-based cohort was reported as 5–7% using the Calin and Berlin criteria. In line with the concept of shared susceptibility and pathophysiology among the spondyloarthritis-related conditions (covered in more detail in Chapter 5), the prevalence of IBP and axSpA are significantly higher in patients with uveitis, psoriasis, or inflammatory bowel disease (IBD) than in the general population. In a secondary care population, the prevalence of IBP, determined using a validated questionnaire, was estimated to be as high as 47%. In a large US population-based study, 31% of people who self-reported psoriasis had chronic back pain, compared to 19% of those not reporting psoriasis. The prevalence of IBP was significantly higher in the psoriasis group (9–17%, depending on which IBP criteria were used) compared with the non-psoriasis group (5–6%). Sacroiliitis is a common incidental finding in patients with IBD undergoing abdominal CT scans, although peripheral joint symptoms are more common than axial symptoms in patients with IBD. In all groups, the presence of back pain was associated with worse quality of life and was higher in those who were also HLA-B27 positive. One study found that in patients with uveitis, significant back pain occurred in 60% of HLA-B27 positive patients, but only in 14% of those who were HLA-B27 negative.

Prevalence of AS, axSpA, and SpA

The global prevalence (frequency of cases in a population) of established AS has been reported to range between 0.01% and 0.2%. There is significant geographic variation in AS, mirroring the differences in HLA-B27 prevalence. The prevalence estimates of AS for each continent have been calculated as 0.07% for Africa, 0.1% for Latin America, 0.17% for Asia, 0.24% for Europe, and 0.32% for North America. It has been calculated that there are approximately 200,000 people with AS in the UK, while approximately 1.30–1.56 million people are thought to have AS in Europe.

Prevalence data for the broader axSpA population is more limited, with US estimates of 0.9–1.4% from a large US study using earlier criteria. Use of the ASAS axSpA classification criteria in epidemiological studies is limited by the requirement for MRI data, which is either absent in population studies or requires studies to be performed in secondary care or high risk populations, leading to selection bias. Studies have estimated a prevalence of axSpA of 0.32–0.7% using the ASAS axSpA criteria. One population-based study has suggested that approximately 20% of patients with axSpA are not diagnosed, so results based solely in secondary care settings are likely to be an underestimation of the prevalence of axSpA. It has been suggested that the total axSpA population is 2–4 times larger than the AS population, which has important implications for healthcare planning and costs.

The global prevalence of combined peripheral and axial spondyloarthritis, defined using older spondyloarthritis (SpA) criteria prior to the ASAS criteria, has been calculated to be around 1%, which would be similar to that for rheumatoid arthritis. There is significant variation between countries and ethnic groups, ranging from 0.01% in Japan up to 2.5% in certain Arctic populations. Much of the variation can be explained by differences in the prevalence of HLA-B27, as well as methodological issues relating to selection bias and the use of classification criteria (developed for use in clinical trials) in epidemiological studies. The only published study to use ASAS criteria estimated the overall prevalence of SpA to be 0.43% of the French population, with 75% of these patients fulfilling the ASAS axSpA criteria and 25% the ASAS peripheral SpA criteria.

Incidence of AS, axSpA, and SpA

The estimates for the incidence (number of new cases in a defined period) of AS range from 0.44 cases per 100,000 person-years in Iceland to 7.3 cases per 100,000 person-years in the USA and northern Norway. It has been calculated that 2,300 new diagnoses of AS are made in the UK each year. The reported incidence estimates for SpA overall range widely from 0.48 (in Japan) to 62.5 (in Spain) cases per 100,000 person years. As before, the wide variations in incidence reflect a combination of genuine geographic and demographic differences as well as methodological differences relating to issues such as sampling and case definition criteria.

Demographics of AS and axSpA

The evolving criteria and disease definitions also impact on the demographics of people classified with these diseases. It is well established that AS, defined by modified New York criteria, commonly presents in the second decade of life and predominantly affects males, at a ratio of 2.5 males: 1 female. In contrast, in nr-axSpA (no x-ray evidence of structural sacroiliac joint damage), the sex distribution is more equally balanced. The implication of this finding could be that either women are genuinely less likely to develop radiographic changes consistent with AS or that women are simply less likely to be diagnosed with the condition due to factors such as low clinical suspicion, concerns about radiographic exposure associated with pelvic x-rays in women, and potential alternative gynaecological causes for back pain.

There also appear to be sex differences between patients fulfilling the clinical and imaging arms of the ASAS axSpA criteria (see Chapter 12). Males make up approximately 60% of the imaging arm (sacroiliitis on x-ray and/or MRI) but only 40% of the clinical arm (no imaging evidence of sacroiliitis). Taken together with accumulating evidence from prospective studies, this suggests that male gender may be associated with increased risk of subsequent radiographic progression.

Not surprisingly, patients with nr-axSpA are more likely to be younger and have shorter disease duration than those with AS. However, nr-axSpA has a similar disease burden to AS, with comparable pain, disease activity, and impact on quality of life (see also Chapter 10). Patients with AS have worse physical function than those with nr-axSpA, presumably reflecting the effects of the longer disease duration and greater spinal radiographic damage.

Natural history and disease progression

By definition, patients with AS already have radiographic evidence of established damage of sacroiliac joints. Despite this, the natural course of radiographic progression is very heterogeneous with significant individual variation. A retrospective cohort indicated that 23% of patients with AS had no evidence of spinal radiographic progression over a mean follow-up of 4 years, while 43% demonstrated significant progression. The only factor in this study to predict radiographic progression was the number of syndesmophytes on baseline x-rays. There was no difference in radiographic progression between genders, but subsequent studies have suggested that smoking and occupational factors are associated with radiographic progression in AS.

The ASAS axSpA criteria (see Chapter 12) were developed in part in response to the recognition that the radiographic changes required to make a diagnosis of definite AS take many years to develop from symptom onset and that there are a significant number of patients with similar symptoms and disease burden who never achieve a formal diagnosis of AS. The underlying assumption and hope was that earlier diagnosis would facilitate earlier treatment, which in turn would lead to better outcomes and prevent or slow progression. This assumption relies on both the expectation that natural progression of the disease will lead to structural damage if untreated and the efficacy of the various therapeutics in preventing disease progression (discussed in more detail in Chapter 15). Data is gradually emerging to suggest that delay in diagnosis is associated with worse outcomes in measures such as disease activity, function, and work impairment, suggesting that earlier intervention would be beneficial for these outcomes. Therefore, a key question for clinicians and funders is whether nr-axSpA represents a prodromal 'early AS' phase with subsequent progression to radiographically evident sacroiliitis. There is now accumulating evidence that a significant number of patients with nr-axSpA do not progress to AS in the short to medium term. Overall, approximately 10% of patients progress from nr-axSpA to AS over 2 years, which has been reported to increase up to 20% over 2 years in the presence of increased C-reactive protein (CRP) levels or inflammatory changes on MRI. Based on data from older studies of 'undifferentiated SpA' in secondary care settings, it had previously been estimated that 10–15% of patients with axSpA will never develop radiographically evident sacroiliitis. However, a recent longstanding population-based cohort in the USA reported that, in fact, only 26% of patients with new-onset nr-axSpA progress to AS over a 15-year period (progression rates at 5 and 10 years follow-up were 6.5% and 18%, respectively). If confirmed, this has important implications for long-term follow-up and monitoring of patients presenting with nr-axSpA. Furthermore, this study indicated that patients in the imaging arm were 3.5 times more likely to progress to AS than subjects in the clinical arm. Therefore, while the clinical features may be similar between these arms, the prognosis differs significantly. The factors that appear to consistently associate with radiographic progression are male gender, high CRP, and positive MRI sacroiliac changes at baseline. These and other observations have raised questions about the performance of the ASAS classification criteria in clinical practice, so steps are underway to improve their validity (see Chapter 12 for more details about the differences between classification and diagnostic criteria). Ultimately it is hoped that clinical, imaging, and/or molecular biomarkers will in future allow better and earlier identification of patients who are at particularly high or low risk of radiographic progression, in order to maximize resource utilization.

Key References and further reading

Stolwijk C, van Onna M, Boonen A, van Tubergen A. The global prevalence of spondyloarthritis: A systematic review and meta-regression analysis. *Arthritis Care Res.* 2015 doi: 10.1002/acr.22831. [Epub ahead of print]

Van Tubergen A. The changing clinical picture and epidemiology of spondyloarthritis. *Nat Rev Rheumatol* 2015;**11**:110–18. doi: 10.1038/nrrheum.2014.181.

Wang R, Gabriel SE, Ward MM. Progression of patients with non-radiographic axial spondyloarthritis to ankylosing spondylitis: a population-based cohort study. *Arthritis Rheumatol* 2016; **68**:1415–21 doi: 10.1002/art.39542.

Chapter 4

The genetics of axial spondyloarthritis

Key points

- Family and twin studies have long suggested a large genetic component in ankylosing spondylitis (AS).
- The genetic association with HLA-B27 remains one of the strongest single gene variant associations reported in any complex polygenic disease.
- The exact mechanism by which HLA-B27 contributes to AS remains unknown, with three main theories proposed: the arthritogenic peptide, endoplasmic reticulum stress with unfolded protein response, and homodimerization theories.
- Genome-wide association studies have identified a number of other important susceptibility genes for AS, several of which overlap with other spondyloarthritis conditions.

Family and twin studies have demonstrated that susceptibility to ankylosing spondylitis (AS) is largely genetically determined with several genetic loci involved. Family and modelling studies have indicated that heritability contributes more than 90% to the overall susceptibility of developing AS. The remaining contribution is due to environmental effects which are likely to be widespread (such as microbiome and biomechanics) rather than limited to those people with the disease.

The majority of the genetic studies to date have been performed in patients with the narrower definition of AS, rather than the wider and more heterogeneous axial spondyloarthritis (axSpA) group. The strongest genetic association with AS is HLA-B27 which was first reported independently by two groups in 1973 (Brewerton, 1973; Schlosstein, 1973). This remains one of the strongest single gene variant associations reported in any complex polygenetic condition. However, despite the strong association and its important role in AS, HLA-B27 only accounts for a minority of the overall genetic susceptibility to AS. Following the description of the association with HLA-B27, there was relatively limited progress in identifying other associated genes until the development of high-throughput sequencing technologies. These technologies facilitated genome-wide association studies (GWAS) which have increased the known loci associated with AS to more than 40. The role and importance of many of these loci are yet to be determined.

HLA-B27

In Caucasian populations, HLA-B27 has a prevalence of 80–90% in those with AS compared to a background population prevalence of 4–7%. While the association of HLA-B27 with AS is found in most ethnic groups, there is significant variation across populations, with the weakest association in those with sub-Saharan African ancestry. HLA-B27 is also associated with related spondyloarthritis (SpA) conditions such as reactive arthritis (70%), psoriatic arthritis with axial involvement (~60%), and acute anterior uveitis (50%). There are over 50 subtypes of HLA-B27, whose evolution and geographical variation largely reflects the migration of humans from Africa. Not all subtypes are associated with AS and some even appear to be protective.

It should be noted that as HLA-B27 occurs in a significant percentage of the population, only a minority of these people will develop AS (less than 10%), although 20% of HLA-B27-positive relatives of patients with AS will develop the condition. Overall, HLA-B27 explains only about 40–50% of the risk for SpA. Therefore, in itself, HLA-B27 is not diagnostic and only reflects an increased susceptibility to develop AS. HLA-B27 status is, therefore, only of relevance in the context of patients with suggestive clinical features (e.g. inflammatory back pain, uveitis). The association of HLA-B27 with peripheral arthritis is low, so checking HLA-B27 is likely to be of more limited clinical value in patients without any axial features (e.g. suggestive axial symptoms or MRI findings), although the 2011 Assessment of SpondyloArthritis international Society (ASAS) classification criteria for peripheral SpA include HLA-B27 as a parameter. The role of HLA-B27 in the classification and diagnosis of AS and axSpA is covered in more detail in Chapter 12.

HLA-B27 is a major histocompatibility complex (MHC) class I molecule involved in antigen presentation, so studies investigating the potential pathogenic role of HLA-B27 in AS initially focused mainly on antigen presentation. Interestingly, HLA-B27-positive individuals are more resistant to certain viral infections, including HIV, hepatitis C, and influenza.

However, despite extensive investigation, the exact mechanism by which HLA-B27 contributes to AS remains unknown. There are currently three major theories proposed to explain how HLA-B27 contributes to the pathophysiology of AS:

1. **Arthritogenic peptide theory**

   This theory proposes that HLA-B27 presents self-peptide complexes to the immune system, thereby eliciting an autoreactive inflammatory response. However, to date, no arthritogenic peptides have been identified, while disease in HLA-B27 animal models of SpA has been shown to be mediated by CD4+ (helper) and not CD8+ (cytotoxic) T cells.

2. **Endoplasmic reticulum stress and unfolded protein response theory**

   This theory proposes that HLA-B27 chains fold more slowly, thereby misfolding and remaining in the endoplasmic reticulum for longer. This, in turn, is proposed to result in endoplasmic reticulum stress and precipitate the pro-inflammatory unfolded protein response in an attempt at homeostasis. Recent data has, however, raised doubt about the endoplasmic reticulum stress and unfolded protein response model in AS.

3. **Homodimerization theory**

   HLA-B27 heavy chains have a propensity to self-associate and homodimerize, resulting in the expression of homodimers on the cell surface which can be recognized by receptors on Th17 and natural killer cells, resulting in IL-17 production.

Other genes implicated in AS susceptibility

GWAS and other studies have identified a number of other genes associated with AS (the key genes are shown in Table 4.1). Other MHC genes (such as HLA-B60) have been implicated but in many cases these have been confounded by linkage to HLA-B27 or not been replicated in other cohorts.

Many of the genes identified in associated with AS can be grouped into one of several overlapping mechanistic pathways (see Box 4.1), with the most notable pathways including:

1. innate immunity—e.g. interleukin (IL)-1, IL-1 receptor
2. antigen-presentation—e.g. HLA-B27, ERAP1 and 2
3. Th17 pathway—e.g. IL-23 receptor, IL-12β

Not all patients with axSpA develop ankylosis, but to date, no genes have been consistently identified that are associated with the ankylosis process, although a few potential candidates have been observed in certain populations, but not subsequently replicated (e.g. *ANTXR2*).

Table 4.1 Key susceptibility genes in ankylosing spondylitis

Gene name	Description
HLA-B27	Human leucocyte antigen; major histocompatibility complex, class I, B
HLA-B60	Human leucocyte antigen; major histocompatibility complex, class I, B
IL-23R	Interleukin 23 receptor
ERAP1	Endoplasmic reticulum aminopeptidase 1
ERAP2	Endoplasmic reticulum aminopeptidase 2
IL12B	Interleukin 12B
IL6R	Interleukin 6 receptor
RUNX3	Runt-related transcription factor
TNFRSF1A	Tumor-necrosis factor-receptor superfamily member 1A
IL1R1-IL1R2 locus	Interleukin 1 receptor
TBkBP1	TNFR-associated factor family member-associated nuclear factor-κB-binding kinase 1-binding protein
KIF21B	Kinesin family member 21B
2p15	Intergenic region (no translated gene product encoded)
21q22	Intergenic region (no translated gene product encoded)
LNPEP	Leucyl/cystinyl aminopeptidase
NPEPPS	Aminopeptidase puromycin-sensitive
TYK2	Tyrosine kinase 2
CARD9	Caspase recruitment-domain family member 9
GPR35	G-protein-coupled receptor 35
GPR65	G-protein-coupled receptor 65
PTGER4	prostaglandin E receptor 4
IL7R	Interleukin 7 receptor
UBE2E3	Ubiquitin-conjugating enzyme E2 E3
UBE2L3	Ubiquitin-conjugating enzyme E2 L3

Box 4.1 Potential pathways or roles of susceptibility genes identified in ankylosing spondylitis

Antigen presentation or processing

HLA-B27, ERAP1, ERAP2, LNPEP, NPEPPS

Th17 and IL-23/IL-17 pathway

IL-23R, IL12B, TYK2, IL6, (TNFRSF1A)

Innate immunity

IL1R1-IL1R2 locus, *(CARD9, TBkBP1)*

Ubiquitination

UBE2E3, UBE2L3

Lymphocyte development

RUNX3, IL7R

G-protein coupled receptors

GPR35, GPR65, (PTGER4)

Intergenic regions with no translated gene product (gene and role unknown)

2p15, 21q22

Interestingly, the implicated pathways, and several of the implicated genes, have also been reported to be associated with the clinically related conditions psoriasis, psoriatic arthritis, and Crohn's disease (see Chapter 8 on extra-articular manifestations of axSpA). Therefore, there appear to be gene associations that are shared between these conditions (e.g. *IL23R, ERAP1*) and other associations that are more disease-specific (e.g. *HLA-B27* in AS, *NOD2* in Crohn's disease). The genetics, therefore, lend further support to the clinical concept of SpA and help explain why many patients have overlapping clinical features. Furthermore, the genetics suggest there are shared pathogenetic mechanisms, in addition to disease-specific processes, which has important therapeutic implications. In particular, the significant number of shared variants between AS and inflammatory bowel disease (IBD) lends support to the hypothesis that gut involvement is an important contributor to the development of AS in a significant number of patients. It seems likely that combinatorial assortments of multiple variants may dictate the pathological outcome, helping to explain how shared pathways lead to the development of different and heterogeneous diseases.

A few of the more recently described non-MHC genes have been studied in more detail and are worthy of further comment.

ERAP1 and 2

Endoplasmic reticulum aminopeptidase (ERAP) 1 was identified by GWAS as being strongly associated with AS, second only to HLA-B27. *ERAP1* has been calculated to contribute about 25% of the risk for AS. Subsequently ERAP2, a structurally and functionally related aminopeptidase, was also found to be associated with AS. The associations with ERAP1 and 2 are especially relevant as they act in the same pathogenic pathway as HLA-B27, suggesting functional importance. Furthermore, ERAP 1 and 2 have been shown to genetically and functionally interact with HLA-B27. Interestingly, *ERAP1* alleles are only associated with AS if HLA-B27 is also present, while *ERAP2* variants are associated with HLA-B27-negative cases. The interaction of *ERAP1* and *HLA-B27* represents the first described true gene–gene interaction in any disease.

ERAP1 and 2 have also been shown to be associated with various other SpA-related conditions, IBD, psoriasis, anterior uveitis, and juvenile enthesitis-associated arthritis, adding further support to their key role in these conditions. Interestingly, in common with HLA-B27, ERAP1 and 2 are also associated with resistance to HIV infection.

ERAP1 functions as a molecular ruler which trims peptides to their optimal length for presentation on MHC-I. Therefore, ERAP1 variants could lead to anomalous peptides of incorrect length or sequence, or altered rates of peptide trimming. While *ERAP1* polymorphisms can potentially contribute to all three theories proposed for HLA-B27's role in AS, the presentation of arthritogenic peptides due to altered peptide trimming is particularly appealing. Determining the exact role of individual *ERAP1* variants in AS is complicated by the presence of multiple *ERAP1* variants in the same patient, so the observed AS phenotype is likely to be a net result of multiple single nucleotide polymorphisms (SNPs), rather than due to a single variant. It is now clear that some *ERAP1* variants increase susceptibility to AS, while others are protective.

Two other aminopeptidases (*LNPEP* and *NPEPPS)* are also associated with AS, further adding to the complexity of understanding the effect of individual variants, but also highlighting the importance of antigen presentation in the pathogenesis of AS.

IL-23 receptor (IL-23R) and IL-23-related genes

The *IL23R* locus has been found to be associated with several of the SpA conditions, including AS, psoriasis, and IBD, although this association is not found in all populations. The association with *IL23R* is of particular interest with the description of IL-23R positive T cells in the entheseal region of SpA animal models (covered in more detail in the pathogenesis section in Chapter 5) and the development of effective agents that target the IL-23/17 pathway. A number of other genes relating to the IL-23/17 pathway have also been identified as susceptibility genes in AS, supporting the importance of this pathway in AS and related SpA conditions. In addition to *IL23R*, these genes include *IL12B, TYK2, IL6R*, and *IL27*.

However, understanding the therapeutic implications of susceptibility genes identified by GWAS is not without challenge, as demonstrated by *IL6R*. This gene has been identified and confirmed by GWAS studies as a susceptibility gene for AS, but in clinical trials, the anti-IL-6R antibodies tocilizumab and sarilumab did not improve clinical outcomes in AS, despite reducing CRP levels. Therapies targeting IL-23 and IL-17 are addressed in the section on pharmacological therapies (Chapter 15).

In summary, despite the strong heritability of AS and significant progress in identifying the susceptibility genes, this is a complex, multigenic disease where different combinations of risk loci interact with each other and with environmental and other factors to yield the clinical phenotype observed in an individual patient.

Furthermore, in addition to disease-associated SNP variants identified by GWAS, there may also be variations in epigenetics, deletions, and copy number which contribute to AS susceptibility and further complicate the picture. The genetic discoveries are, however, yielding important clues regarding the underlying biology of AS which should lead to further therapeutic, diagnostic and prognostic advances in future.

It should be noted that the effect sizes of individual susceptibility loci identified in GWAS studies are relatively low, so routine genetic testing beyond HLA-B27 in clinical practice cannot currently be justified. The role of HLA-B27 in the diagnostic process is covered in more detail in the classification section (Chapter 12).

Key References and further reading

Brewerton DA, Hart FD, Nicholls A *et al.* Ankylosing spondylitis and HLA 27. *Lancet.* 1973;1(7809):904–7. doi: 10.1016/S0140-6736(73)92026-6

Reveille J. Genetics of spondyloarthritis—beyond the MHC. *Nat Rev Rheum.* 2012;**8**(5):296–304. doi: 10.1038/nrrheum.2012.41

Schlosstein LH, Terasaki PI, Bluestone R, Pearson CM. High association of an HL-A antigen, W27, with ankylosing spondylitis. *N Engl J Med.* 1973;**288**(14):704–6. doi: 10.1056/NEJM197304052881403.

Tsui FW, Tsui HW, Akram *et al.* The genetic basis of ankylosing spondylitis: new insights into disease pathogenesis. *Appl Clinc Genet.* 2014;7:105–15. doi: 10.2147/TACG.S37325

Chapter 5

The pathophysiology and immunology of axial spondyloarthritis

Key points

- Ankylosing spondylitis (AS) is a heterogeneous and complex disease. While the exact pathophysiology remains unclear, significant advances have recently been made in the understanding of several implicated processes.
- Genetic and pathophysiological studies implicate alterations in antigen presentation, innate immunity, the interleukin (IL)-23/IL-17 pathway, microbiome, and biomechanics.
- The pathophysiology of AS appears to represent a complex combination of several processes. The interactions and relative importance of these remain important areas of active ongoing study.
- Overall, the existing evidence suggests that a genetically predisposed host reacts to a dysbiotic process and/or biomechanical stress, altering the immune balance from homeostasis towards a pro-inflammatory state dominated by IL-23/IL-17 activation leading to the clinical phenotype.
- The exact contribution and timing of these events vary between individuals, so understanding this has important implications for future stratified precision medicine in axSpA.

Although the key role of HLA-B27 in ankylosing spondylitis (AS) was identified in the 1970s, the pathophysiology of AS remained unclear and poorly understood until recently. Therefore, many of the initial synthetic and biologic therapies for AS were adopted from rheumatoid arthritis (RA) where the pathophysiology is far better studied and understood. With the development of large genome wide association studies (GWAS) and advances in laboratory techniques, it has become increasingly clear that while AS and RA share common pro-inflammatory pathways (including TNFα), there are significant differences in pathophysiology which are now being exploited to develop novel therapies for AS and axial spondyloarthritis (axSpA). In fact, AS pathophysiology has significant overlap with the related conditions psoriasis, psoriatic arthritis, and inflammatory bowel disease (IBD), leading to sharing of therapies across this spectrum of diseases.

AS is a heterogeneous and complex disease involving a number of processes. Genetic and pathophysiological studies, coupled with the increasingly recognized overlap with other spondyloarthritis (SpA) conditions, implicate alterations in antigen presentation, innate immunity, the interleukin (IL)-23/IL-17 pathway, microbiome, and biomechanics.

HLA-B27, ERAP1, and antigen presentation

The exact mechanism by which HLA-B27 contributes to the pathophysiology of AS remains unknown. The discovery of associations with other susceptibility genes involved in antigen presentation, and in particular the gene–gene interaction with *ERAP1* (see Chapter 4), has led to a renewed surge of interest and research activity in this area. These genetics strongly point to involvement of dysfunctional antigen presentation in the development of AS. The current main theories proposed for the pathogenic mechanisms of HLA-B27 in AS are covered in more detail in the section on the genetics of AS (Chapter 4). Briefly, these include the arthritogenic peptide, endoplasmic reticulum stress with unfolded protein response, and homodimerization theories.

Innate immunity and microbiome

It has long been proposed that intestinal microorganisms may be involved in the development of AS, although the exact mechanisms remain elusive. Up to 8% of patients with AS develop overt IBD, while more than 60% of patients with AS have been found to have microscopic signs of gut inflammation, often without significant gastrointestinal symptoms (Mielants, 1995). Further epidemiologic evidence implicating gut microorganisms and inflammation is provided by the established role of infectious diarrhoea in reactive arthritis and the occurence of inflammatory arthritis in patients with IBD (enteropathic-associated arthritis). In the past, the focus was mainly on identifying specific pathogenic bacteria in AS. However, despite some initial tantalizing leads, this strategy failed to consistently identify any specific pathologic bacteria. It is, however, worth recalling that the commonly used drug sulfasalazine was initially designed to combine an antibacterial agent with salicylate.

The development of culture-independent high-throughput microbial DNA sequencing has led to an exponential advance in the understanding of mucosal immunity, and the bidirectional interaction between microbes and their human hosts. It is now appreciated that the intestinal microbiome helps shape the human immune system, leading to homeostasis in health states or inflammation when dysfunction of the microbiome (dysbiosis) occurs. Dysbiosis has subsequently been implicated in the pathogenesis of a variety of inflammatory rheumatic conditions, with SpA conditions at the forefront due to the clinically evident links with mucosal inflammation. Many of the initial microbiome studies in autoimmune diseases were understandably performed in IBD, which is characterized by a decrease in 'beneficial' intestinal microbiota diversity and an increase in enterobacteria.

The dysbiosis concept is further supported by animal models of SpA, which fail to develop when the animals are raised under germ-free conditions. Gut bacteria are, therefore, a requirement for SpA inflammation in these animal models. Despite the established association of AS with both clinical and microscopic subclinical gut inflammation, relatively few studies have characterized the intestinal microbiome in AS to date. One study reported a higher prevalence of sulfate-reducing bacteria, while another study demonstrated a distinct gut microbial signature in patients with AS.

Interestingly, broad-spectrum antibiotics have not demonstrated efficacy in rheumatic diseases and, in fact, use of antibiotics at a young age has been found to be associated with the subsequent development of a number of inflammatory conditions. Attempts to modulate the composition of intestinal bacteria or their byproducts in order to reduce inflammatory responses are currently underway. Fecal microbial transplantation has proven highly effective in the treatment of severe *Clostridium difficile* colitis and is now being applied to a number of autoimmune conditions, including IBD. This process has outstanding challenges, and careful rigorous study is required to understand whether this approach could be safely adapted for the treatment of SpA.

Despite these significant advances, there remains much to be learned about the role of the microbiome in AS and other rheumatic diseases before intestinal microbiome targeting strategies can become a reality. It remains unclear whether associations with disease states depend on the relative presence or absence of specific classes of microorganisms *per se* or whether they relate more to the presence of certain bacterial components, byproducts, or metabolites. Many of the initial microbiome sequencing studies were limited in utility by methodological issues that are gradually being addressed and standardized. It also remains challenging to determine whether dysbiosis associated with a particular disease is causal or, in fact, an effect of the disease or the immunomodulatory drugs used to treat that disease. Recent literature in IBD also suggests a potential role for the intestinal virome, which has not been evaluated in AS yet, but may be of relevance in light of the known protective role of HLA-B27 in a number of viral infections.

Biomechanics

It has long been recognized that many of the musculoskeletal features of AS and SpA occur at sites of biomechanical stress. Sacroiliac joints, the hallmark site of AS involvement, are joined by several ligaments and are prone to significant mechanical stresses. The vertebral corner lesions, and subsequent syndesmophytes, in the spine also occur at key musculoskeletal attachment sites. Classic sites peripherally include the entheseal insertions of the Achilles tendon and plantar fascia. This enthesitis picture in SpA differs from the situation in RA where systemic inflammation and synovitis dominate, although the latter may also be observed in AS and SpA. The entheses are subjected to repetitive biomechanical stresses during the course of normal muscle, ligament, and tendon actions. These and other observations led to the enthesitis-based model of SpA pathogenesis. An elegant study demonstrated that in a TNF-dependent mouse model, the development of enthesitis and subsequent new bone formation are dependent on continuous biomechanical strain (Jacques, 2013). None of the mice whose hind legs were 'unloaded' by being suspended by their tails, developed hind leg arthritis while all the weight-bearing control mice developed severe enthesitis. How best to address the issue of biomechanical stress as potential trigger of AS is not clear in clinical practice, but requires further study as this has implications for how and when best to deliver physical therapy interventions in these conditions.

The discovery of IL-23 receptor (IL-23R) positive T cells in entheseal sites of a different mouse model, which develops enthesitis in response to overexpression of IL-23, suggests that not only can mechanical stresses trigger inflammatory responses, but that systemic IL-23 can lead to inflammation at these sites. There may therefore be several pathways that lead to enthesitis. Taken together, these data suggest that, in the presence of appropriate genetic and other susceptibility factors, interactions between biomechanical forces and immune responses may lead to disease. The susceptibility factors may include mucosal (such as alterations in the gut microbiome) and systemic (such as IL-23/IL-17) immune factors.

Interestingly, erosions appear to preferentially occur at sites undergoing compression, whereas new bone formation occurs mainly at sites subject to tensile forces.

Cytokines in AS

Tumour necrosis factor (TNF)

TNF has been found to be overexpressed in the circulation, synovial fluid, and target tissue (sacroiliac and facet joints) in patients with AS, while the phenotypes of several animal models overexpressing TNF more closely resemble SpA than RA. The efficacy of TNF inhibitors in patients with AS and axSpA further supports the involvement of TNF in the pathophysiology of AS. However, it should be noted that TNF is also produced by certain T cells in response to IL-23, so this is entirely compatible with the central role of the IL-23/IL-17 pathway (described later in this chapter). In fact, the TNF inhibitors may be exerting many of their beneficial effects in AS by inhibiting this pathway.

The relationship between inflammation and new bone formation in AS remains unclear, particularly in the context of TNF. TNF is an important inducer of osteoclast activity and excess TNF activity leads to erosive disease, as observed in RA. TNF blockers strongly retard or even arrest structural damage in RA, but initial studies suggested this was not the case in AS, with evidence of radiographic progression, despite clinical response and reduction in inflammation. In contrast to RA, in AS there is not only bony loss, but also new bone formation in the form of syndesmophytes/enthesiophytes which over time can lead to ankylosis. MRI studies have shown that active corner inflammatory lesions predict the development of syndesmophytes. One possible explanation for the apparent lack of radiographic response with TNF inhibitors is that there may be persistent mild inflammation not detected by MRI or other means, which leads to ongoing radiographic progression. However, the recognition that syndesmophytes were more likely to develop at the sites of resolved corner inflammatory lesions rather than sites of persistent lesions, led to the 'TNF brake' hypothesis. This hypothesis suggests that while there is ongoing active inflammation, TNF suppresses new bone formation, via a number of regulatory pathways, but that when inflammation resolves (e.g. in response to treatment with TNF inhibitors), the brake is released, allowing tissue repair and new bone formation to occur. As a result of this uncoupling between inflammation and new bone formation, patients who otherwise respond well to anti-TNF therapy may appear to have radiographic progression due to the new bone formation (which would have occurred in many anyway, but at a later date, in the absence of TNF inhibition). Additional research is needed to confirm whether progression is due to persistent, low-grade inflammation or to the release of the TNF brake once inflammation is effectively treated, but there is accumulating data to suggest that when patients are followed up for longer, treatment with TNF blockers results in slowing of radiographic progression, supporting the latter mechanism. There is much ongoing active research in the area of osteoimmunology, which is beyond the scope of this publication, but which may yield novel future therapeutic targets to directly target bone involvement in AS.

The IL-23/IL-17 axis

In addition to confirming the importance of HLA-B27 and ERAP1 in AS, the GWAS studies also indicated that AS shares key cytokine pathways with psoriasis and IBD (see also Chapter 4). Many of the lessons being learned in these conditions, and subsequent development of therapies for these conditions, are now being tested in AS and are likely to reach the clinic shortly.

Investigating the immunology of AS is complicated by difficulty accessing the target tissue (entheses or spine) in humans. Therefore, much of the current state of knowledge is based on information from the human GWAS studies, animal models, and by measuring circulating cytokine levels. It should be noted that each of these methodologies has their weaknesses: the genetics mainly indicate susceptibility; animal models cannot fully reflect the complexity in humans and are not subject to the same environmental and biomechanical forces; and circulating cytokine levels fluctuate and may not accurately reflect the situation in the target tissues. However, despite this, these studies provide compelling evidence implicating the IL-23/IL-17 pathway in the pathogenesis of AS and the related SpA conditions. The importance of this pathway is further supported by recent therapeutic trials reporting clinically relevant benefits by inhibiting IL-17 and IL-23.

The longstanding T helper (Th) cell paradigm that naive T cells differentiate into either Th1 or Th2 cells was dramatically changed by the discovery of Th17, and subsequently other Th subtypes. This paradigm shift challenged many of the traditional autoimmune disease models. In response to pro-inflammatory cytokines, such as IL-1, IL-6, and IL-23, and activation of the transcription factor STAT3, naive CD4+ T cells differentiate into Th17 cells. It has subsequently been shown that Th17 cells themselves are heterogeneous and there is an emerging view that local cytokines and conditions influence the precise T-cell phenotype. These Th17 cells in turn express the transcription factor RORγt and produce the cytokine IL-17.

Th17 cells express IL-23R on their surface and IL-23 is essential for the differentiation and proliferation of Th17 cells, as well as maintenance of IL-17 production. GWAS studies have identified variants of the *IL23R* gene in association with AS, as well as IBD and psoriasis, implicating *IL23R* as a common susceptibility factor across the SpA spectrum. Subsequently, several other genes whose products may influence IL-23 and Th17 development have been identified in association with AS, including *TYK2, STAT3, IL12B*, and *IL6R*. The gene *IL12B* encodes IL-12p40, the common subunit of IL-12 and IL-23, which is targeted by the monoclonal antibody ustekinumab used in clinic for the treatment of psoriasis, psoriatic arthritis, and IBD, and which is currently undergoing trials in AS. The convergence of these gene products in the IL-23/IL-17 axis strongly implicates this pathway in the pathogenesis of AS and SpA conditions.

IL-17 consists of six family members, with IL-17A the best studied and the target of many of the initial anti-IL-17 therapies. IL-17A has multiple biologic effects, including induction of the key pro-inflammatory cytokines IL-6 and TNF. The physiological roles of IL-17 include host defence against extracellular bacterial and fungal pathogens, as well as some intracellular pathogens. Recent evidence also suggests that IL-17 helps maintain integrity of the intestinal barrier.

It has subsequently been recognized that most of the IL-17 is, in fact, produced by an expanding range of innate immune cells, which include but are not limited to γδ T cells, neutrophils, and a range of natural killer cells, rather than by actual Th17 T cells. In common with Th17 cells, most of these cells are activated by IL-23, which is produced by dendritic cells and macrophages exposed to microbial products. This provides an appealing potential link between IL-17 production and the alterations in gut or skin microbiome and permeability that are observed in axSpA and SpA conditions.

In addition to IL-17, Th17 cells also produce other cytokines, including TNF, IL-6, IL-22 and IL-21. Interestingly, IL-22 may promote osteoproliferation, while IL-17 (and TNF) lead to bone loss, so the combination of these cytokines may help explain some of the apparently paradoxical combination of bone loss and osteoproliferation in patients with AS or psoriatic arthritis. The mechanisms that determine which of these processes dominate at a particular site are not understood, but are likely to relate to local conditions and cytokine levels.

Dysregulation of the IL-23/IL-17 axis in patients with AS has been reported in an increasing number of studies, further supporting the importance of this pathway in AS. A full review of these studies is beyond the scope of this publication, so only key factors are covered here. Patients with active AS and psoriatic arthritis have increased levels of IL-17 and IL-23 in serum and synovial fluid. As is often the case for circulating cytokines, correlations with disease activity or severity have been variable and inconsistent. Increasing numbers of circulating Th17 T cells, particularly KIR3DL2+ CD4+ T cells, have also been reported in serum and synovial fluid of patients with AS. Importantly, increased expression of IL-17 and IL-23 has been documented in various cell types, including innate immune cells, at sites of inflammation such as synovium and facet joints. Furthermore, there appears to be a correlation with genetic variants; patients with the protective *IL23R* variant were associated with decreased expression of Th17 genes, while patients with greater numbers of SNPs on the IL-23/IL-17 pathway had higher levels of Th17-associated mRNA.

Observations in HLA-B27 transgenic rats indicate that the SpA-like picture observed in this animal model is mediated by CD4+ (helper) rather than CD8+ (cytotoxic) T cells. In this rat model, classic CD8+ T cell recognition of HLA-B27 is not required for the SpA-like features, while overexpression of HLA-B27 alone is sufficient to result in CD4+ Th17 activation. It has been postulated that this activation of Th17 may occur by HLA-B27 misfolding leading to endoplasmic reticulum stress or due to homodimerization of HLA-B27. Interestingly, inflammation of the gut in these rats occurs very early and is dependent on gut flora, raising the possibility that changes in the gut microbiome may influence IL-23/IL-17 pathway activation.

An important advance in understanding and linking the various immunological postulates in SpA was the identification of a previously unrecognized population of IL23R-expressing T cells in the entheses and other key SpA-related sites of mice (Sherlock, 2012). When IL-23 was systemically overexpressed in these previously healthy mice, this resulted in local expression of IL-17, TNFα, and IL-22 associated with entheseal inflammation (enthesitis) at peripheral and axial sites, and subsequent IL-22-dependent new bone formation. Furthermore, TNF inhibition resulted in significantly less reduction in this IL-23 driven enthesitis, compared with IL-17 and IL-22 inhibition, particularly when the latter two were administered in combination. This study has significant implications as it potentially starts to unite many of the previously apparently disparate strands of gut inflammation, HLA-B27, IL-23/IL-17 involvement, and enthesitis, although this has yet to be confirmed in humans. This study also implies AS can develop independently of any tissue- or organ-specific autoreactivity.

While in humans TNFα is mainly implicated in synovitis and erosions (as seen in RA), the pathologic situation in SpA is likely to be a complex combination and interplay of TNF, IL-17, IL-22, and IL-23. Understanding the relative importance and hierarchy of these processes in different individuals and tissues, and at different time-points in the disease, will be crucial for the optimal use of biologic therapies in axSpA.

Summary

Therefore, the pathophysiology of AS appears to represent a complex combination of several processes. The interactions and relative importance of these remain important areas of active ongoing study. Overall, the existing evidence suggests that a genetically predisposed host reacts to a dysbiotic process and/or biomechanical stress, altering the immune balance from homeostasis towards a pro-inflammatory state dominated by IL-23/IL-17 activation leading to the clinical phenotype. The exact contribution and timing of these events is likely to vary between individuals, so understanding this has important implications for future stratified precision medicine in axSpA.

Key References and further reading

Jacques P, Lambrecht S, Verheugen E *et al.* Proof of concept: enthesitis and new bone formation in spondyloarthritis are driven by mechanical strain and stromal cells. *Ann Rheum Dis.* 2014;**73**:437–45. doi: 10.1136/annrheumdis-2013-2039243

Mielants H, Veys EM, Cuvelier C, *et al.* The evolution of spondyloarthropathies in relation to gut histology. II. Histological aspects. *J Rheumatol.* 1995;**22**(12):2273–8. PMID: 8835561

Scher JU, Littman DR, Abramson SB. Microbiome in inflammatory arthritis and human rheumatic diseases. *Arthritis Rheumatol.* 2016;**68**(1):35–45. doi: 10.1002/art.39259.

Sherlock JP, Joyce-Shaikh B, Turner SP, *et al.* IL-23 induces spondyloarthropathy by acting on ROR-γt+ CD3+CD4-CD8- entheseal resident T cells. *Nat Med.* 2012;**18**(7):1069–76. doi: 10.1038/nm.2817.

Smith JA, Colbert RA. The interleukin-23/interleukin-17 axis in spondyloarthritis pathogenesis: Th17 and beyond. *Arthritis Rheumatol.* 2014;**66**(2):231–41. doi: 10.1002/art.38291.

Chapter 6

Inflammatory back pain

Key points

- Inflammatory back pain (IBP) refers to a collection of symptoms that help identify patients with possible inflammatory spinal disease.
- Symptoms suggestive of IBP include: onset of symptoms aged <40 years, improvement with exercise, worsening with rest, early morning stiffness lasting >30 minutes, and improvement with NSAIDs.
- IBP criteria were initially developed and validated in patients with ankylosing spondylitis, but have subsequently been shown to perform similarly in patients with axial spondyloarthritis (axSpA).
- The Berlin criteria demonstrated the highest specificity (84%) and the Calin criteria the highest sensitivity (92%) for axSpA.
- IBP does not equate to axSpA but should raise the possibility and trigger appropriate referral or investigation.

Chronic back pain is the commonest presenting feature in axial spondyloarthritis (axSpA). However, chronic back pain is extremely common and only a small fraction of people with this symptom will have axSpA (see Chapter 3). Some common causes of chronic back pain are listed in Box 6.1, although it should be noted that in most patients it is not possible to identify an exact cause and the term 'non-specific' or 'mechanical' back pain is often used in this setting. Therefore, the challenge in clinical practice is to identify those patients presenting with chronic back pain who are likely to have axSpA.

The concept of inflammatory back pain (IBP) therefore evolved in an effort to help distinguish those with a probable underlying inflammatory cause for their back pain from those with the far more prevalent non-specific mechanical back pain. It is clearly not feasible or desirable to investigate all patients with chronic back pain, so recognizing those

Box 6.1 Potential sources of chronic low back pain

Potential sources of chronic back pain
Non-specific low back pain (no obvious cause)
Degenerative disc disease
Facet joint disease
Muscle or ligament pain
Herniated discs
Spondylolisthesis
Severe kyphosis or scoliosis
Osteoporotic wedge fracture
Spinal stenosis or radiculopathy
Inflammation due to axial spondyloarthritis or related spondyloarthritis conditions
Infections: septic discitis, osteomyelitis, epidural abscess
Tumours: primary or metastases
Abdominal aortic aneurysm
Renal disorders
Endometriosis
Gastrointestinal disorders
Fibromyalgia

with features suggestive of IBP is an important first step in identifying potential patients who may have axSpA. A comparison of symptoms suggestive of mechanical and inflammatory chronic low back pain is shown in Table 6.1.

The first reported description of the typical inflammatory axial symptoms experienced by patients with ankylosing spondylitis (AS) was in 1947 by Hart who documented spinal stiffness, particularly on waking in the morning, with gradual improvement on activity during the day and worsening with inactivity. Since then, a number of different IBP criteria sets have been developed in an attempt to operationalize the identification and measurement of IBP, mainly for epidemiological and clinical research. While the specific features vary across criteria, there are several common features such as relatively young age of onset, duration for at least 3 months, morning stiffness, and improvement with activity. Other suggestive features include insidious onset, pain at night, worsening with rest, and alternating buttock pain.

Table 6.1 Comparison of typical symptoms of chronic mechanical and inflammatory back pain

Mechanical back pain	Inflammatory back pain
Any age of onset	Age at onset typically <40 years
Variable onset; often acute	Insidious onset
Worsens with movement or exercise	Improves with exercise
Often improves with rest	Does not improve with rest
Morning stiffness uncommon; if present then usually lasts for <30 minutes	Morning stiffness usually >30 minutes
May improve in bed at night	Pain at night (may require patient to get up)
Variable response to non-steroidal anti-inflammatory drugs (NSAIDs)	Often good response to NSAIDs
Buttock pain less common (may be referred)	May report alternating buttock pain

Calin Criteria (1977)

The first formal IBP criteria were developed by Calin et al. in 1977 (Calin, 1977). These criteria are fulfilled if four of the following five parameters are present: age at onset <40 years, back pain duration >3 months, insidious onset, morning stiffness, and improvement with exercise (Box 6.2). The

Box 6.2 Calin criteria for inflammatory back pain (Calin, 1977)

Age at onset <40 years
Insidious onset
Back pain persisting >3 months
Morning stiffness
Improvement with exercise

The Calin criteria for IBP are fulfilled if at least four of the five parameters are present (sensitivity 95%, specificity 85%).

Adapted from Calin A, Porta J, Fries JF, et al. Clinical history as a screening test for ankylosing spondylitis. JAMA. 1977;237(24):2613-2614 and Sieper et al. The Assessment of SpondyloArthritis international Society (ASAS) handbook: A guide to assess spondyloarthritis. Ann Rheum Dis. *2009b;68(Suppl II):ii1–44.*

authors reported sensitivity of 95% and specificity of 85% in their test population, although specificity was lower when applied to other populations.

Berlin Criteria (2006)

The Berlin criteria were developed as a result of a study designed to assess the components of IBP, individually and in various combinations, in patients younger than 50 years with low back pain for at least 3 months (Rudwaleit, 2006). Three sets of four variable combinations were defined and found to perform similarly. The authors expressed a preference for the set which was easy to administer in a clinical setting and which had higher specificity than the Calin criteria. These criteria included age of onset of back pain <50 years and duration >3 months as entry criterion plus at least two of the following four criteria: morning stiffness >30 minutes, improvement with exercise but not with rest, awakening in the second half of the night due to back pain, and alternating buttock pain (Box 6.3). The authors reported sensitivity of 70% with specificity of 81% for these criteria.

Box 6.3 Berlin criteria for inflammatory back pain (Rudwaleit, 2006)

Berlin criteria for IBP: to be applied in patients aged <50 years with chronic back pain (>3 months duration)

Morning stiffness of >30 minutes duration

Improvement in back pain with exercise but *not* with rest

Awakening during the second half of the night because of back pain

Alternating buttock pain

The Berlin criteria for IBP are fulfilled if at least two of the four parameters are present.

Adapted from Rudwaleit et al. *Inflammatory back pain in ankylosing spondylitis: a reassessment of the clinical history for application as classification and diagnostic criteria.* Arthritis Rheum. *2006;54(2):569–78 and Sieper* et al. *The Assessment of SpondyloArthritis international Society (ASAS) handbook: a guide to assess spondyloarthritis.* Ann Rheum Dis. *2009b;68(Suppl II):ii1–44*

ASAS IBP according to experts criteria (2009)

The subsequent Assessment of SpondyloArthritis international Society (ASAS) IBP criteria developed from a workshop of international experts convened to develop new classification criteria for spondyloarthritis (Sieper, 2009a). As part of a Delphi exercise, experts made judgements on various IBP parameters based on their evaluation of 20 patients with suspected axSpA.

Box 6.4 ASAS expert criteria for inflammatory back pain (Sieper, 2009a)

ASAS expert criteria for IBP: to be applied in patients with chronic back pain (>3 months duration)

Age at onset < 40 years

Insidious onset

Improvement with exercise

No improvement with rest

Pain at night (with improvement on getting up)

The ASAS expert criteria for IBP are fulfilled if at least four of the five parameters are present.

reproduced from the Annals of Rheumatic Diseases, Sieper et al. *New criteria for inflammatory back pain in patients with chronic back pain: a real patient exercise by experts from the Assessment of SpondyloArthritis international Society (ASAS). Vol 68, Issue 6, 2009 with permission from the BMJ publishing group.*

Analysis of the concordance among experts led to a definition of IBP which required patients with chronic back pain to meet four of the following five criteria: age at onset <40 years, insidious onset, improvement with exercise, no improvement with rest, or nocturnal pain (with improvement on getting up) (Box 6.4). The reported sensitivity for these criteria was 80% with specificity of 72% in a validation cohort. These criteria share many features with the previous IBP criteria. However, as the criteria name suggests, while the earlier criteria were developed by comparing patients with AS to patients with other types of back pain, these criteria were based on the judgement of experts.

Utility of IBP criteria in clinical and research settings

The various IBP criteria were developed and their performance validated in patients with AS, prior to the development of the ASAS classification criteria for axSpA. In a subsequent study comparing the three main IBP criteria in patients with axSpA and mechanical back pain, the Calin criteria had the highest sensitivity (92%) while the Berlin criteria had the highest specificity (84%). The ASAS expert criteria sensitivity and specificity in this study were 77% and 72%, respectively. These results suggest the IBP criteria perform similarly for both AS and axSpA. None of the criteria sets have been validated for patient self-completion, although a preliminary validation of a new self-reported screening questionnaire has been reported. This study observed that the single self-reported item 'diurnal variation', which is implied by references to 'morning stiffness' but not directly incorporated in the existing criteria, demonstrated significant classification utility in patients with axSpA and mechanical back pain in a tertiary rheumatology setting.

Evaluation of the individual IBP components demonstrated that spontaneous awakening in the night with pain, improvement of pain with exercise, and alternating buttock pain performed the best with likelihood ratios of 3.3, 2.1, and 2.2 respectively. The specific details for each individual component of the IBP criteria are also important. Morning stiffness, for example, can be equally present in patients with both mechanical and inflammatory back pain but a cut-off greater than 30 minutes appears to distinguish those with an inflammatory component to their spinal pain.

It has been long recognized that there are many patients in the community with axSpA who remain undiagnosed. Therefore, it had been hoped that, despite being developed as classification criteria, the various IBP criteria could be used to facilitate screening for IBP, particularly in primary care settings. Despite significant efforts to increase the awareness of healthcare professionals about the concept of IBP, knowledge of IBP features remains limited in primary care. A UK study reported that 17% of primary care doctors were able to identify fewer than four features suggestive of IBP, although there is likely to be significant regional and national variation in awareness of IBP in primary care settings. The value of incorporating IBP in referral strategies to promote earlier diagnosis of axSpA has been evaluated in a number of studies. A review of the literature concluded that in a primary care setting, approximately 43% of patients referred with IBP had axSpA, with best performance when IBP was used in combination with other referral parameters such as positive HLA-B27 or imaging evidence of sacroiliitis. The limited value of IBP in primary care settings reflects, in part, the methodology whereby IBP classification criteria were developed in limited and somewhat artificially constructed populations. Furthermore, the sensitivity and specificity of IBP criteria depend on the pre-test probability of the patient having AxSpA, which will vary significantly depending on the local prevalence of axSpA and the clinical setting.

The prevalence of IBP in patients with chronic back pain in primary care in the UK was reported to be 14.7%. In contrast, patients with inflammatory bowel disease and anterior uveitis have a higher pre-test probability, and therefore higher likelihood, of IBP and axSpA. The prevalence of IBP has been reported to be a high as 47% in one study of patients with anterior uveitis attending ophthalmology clinics. Therefore, screening for IBP and axSpA is likely to have greater value and yield in higher risk patients attending gastroenterology, dermatology, and ophthalmology clinics, than in unselected primary care populations.

It should also be noted that while the concept of IBP is used most frequently in the context of AS and axSpA, the presence of positive criteria for IBP does not equate with a diagnosis of these conditions. Importantly, IBP is not a single clinical entity and many patients with apparent IBP will not have axSpA. A large US population cohort study reported prevalence estimates of 5–6% for IBP compared to 1% for SpA. It is still unclear whether IBP represents a precursor to axSpA or is just a descriptive collection of symptoms, although the latter appears more likely. It also still remains to be determined whether treatment of IBP will have long-term or just short-term symptomatic benefits. More recently, rather than having stand-alone IBP criteria, IBP itself has been incorporated into classification criteria for axSpA (covered in more detail in Chapter 12). However, these remain classification criteria rather than diagnostic criteria, so making a diagnosis of axSpA in a patient with IBP relies on the pre-test probability of a diagnosis of axSpA and excluding other potential causes for IBP (this concept is covered in more detail in Chapter 12).

In summary, the concept of IBP is helpful in raising the clinical suspicion for axSpA. Despite the development of a number of IBP classification criteria, these remain of limited value in clinical settings. However, symptoms suggestive of IBP, particularly in combination with other clinical, imaging, and genetic factors, should raise the possibility of a diagnosis of axSpA and trigger appropriate referral or investigation, based on the likelihood of axSpA.

Key References and further reading

Braun A, Saracbasi E, Grifka J, *et al.* Identifying patients with axial spondyloarthritis in primary care: how useful are items indicative of inflammatory back pain? *Ann Rheum Dis.* 2011;**70**(10):1782–7. doi: 10.1136/ard.2011.151167

Calin A, Porta J, Fries JF, *et al.* Clinical history as a screening test for ankylosing spondylitis. *JAMA.* 1977;**237**(24):2613–4. doi:10.1001/jama.1977.03270510035017

Rudwaleit M, Metter A, Listing J, *et al.* Inflammatory back pain in ankylosing spondylitis: a reassessment of the clinical history for application as classification and diagnostic criteria. *Arthritis Rheum.* 2006;**54**(2):569–78. doi: 10.1002/art.21619

Rudwaleit M, van der Heijde D, Landewe R, *et al.* The development of Assessment of SpondyloArthritis international Society classification criteria for axial spondyloarthritis (part II): validation and final selection. *Ann Rheum Dis.* 2009;**68**(6):777–83. doi: 10.1136/ard.2009.108233

Sieper J, van der Heijde D, Landewe R, *et al.* New criteria for inflammatory back pain in patients with chronic back pain: a real patient exercise by experts from the Assessment of SpondyloArthritis international Society (ASAS). *Ann Rheum Dis.* 2009a;**68**(6):784–8. doi: 10.1136/ard.2008.101501

Sieper J, Rudwaleit M, Baraliakos X, *et al.* The Assessment of SpondyloArthritis international Society (ASAS) handbook: a guide to assess spondyloarthritis. *Ann Rheum Dis.* 2009b;**68**(Suppl II):ii1–44. doi: 10.1136/ard.2008.104018.

Chapter 7

Peripheral musculoskeletal involvement in axial spondyloarthritis

Key points

- Many patients with axial spondyloarthritis (axSpA) also develop peripheral musculoskeletal involvement. This can include peripheral joint synovitis, enthesitis, and dactylitis.
- Peripheral musculoskeletal involvement is an important component of the disease with significant impact on function and quality of life.
- Many of the features may be subtle and overlooked, unless specifically evaluated and examined. In particular, hip disease is a bad prognostic feature and, if present, may require more aggressive therapy or surgical intervention.
- On occasion, further imaging may be required to detect enthesitis or subtle joint inflammation in order to inform treatment decisions.

In addition to the axial diseases that characterizes axial spondyloarthritis (axSpA), many patients also develop peripheral musculoskeletal involvement. This can include peripheral joint synovitis, enthesitis, and dactylitis.

Peripheral arthritis

Patients with axSpA may develop an asymmetric, oligoarticular inflammatory arthritis. On occasion, peripheral joint involvement can be the first presentation, so patients with a suggestive joint distribution and/or with other features suggestive of spondyloarthritis (SpA) (e.g. family history, inflammatory bowel disease), should be specifically asked about axial symptoms suggestive of inflammatory back pain (see Chapter 6). The most commonly affected joints are the larger joints of the lower limbs (ankles and knees), as well as the shoulders. Smaller joint involvement can also be seen, with some patients developing symmetric polyarthritis, although this is uncommon and usually occurs later in the disease when the diagnosis is already known.

The prevalence of peripheral arthritis has been estimated to be between 15–55%, depending on the type of cohort and whether the presence of peripheral arthritis is defined clinically or radiologically. In a German inception cohort of patients with axSpA, peripheral arthritis was noted in 14% of subjects with ankylosing spondylitis (AS), and 18% in subjects with non-radiographic axSpA (nr-axSpA) (Rudwaleit, 2009). In a French cohort of patients with early inflammatory low back pain, the prevalence of peripheral arthralgia was 53%, with synovitis in 22% of those patients fulfilling the modified New York criteria for AS (Dougados, 2011). In a recent large multinational cross-sectional study, peripheral articular involvement was reported in 56% of 4000 patients with SpA, although this included patients fulfilling both the axial and peripheral ASAS criteria (Moltó, 2016).

It is unclear why larger joints closer to the axial skeleton (or 'root joints') are more frequently involved compared to more appendicular joints. Some researchers have hypothesized that mechanical loading and physical strain on these weight-bearing joints can act as a trigger for inflammation, but this has not been confirmed.

If involved, the peripheral joints can display synovitis, entheseal inflammation (enthesitis), and bone marrow involvement. In contrast to the purely osteodestructive and erosive changes seen in rheumatoid arthritis (RA), a combination of osteolytic and osteoproliferative processes may occur concurrently in axSpA. Therefore, patients may have a combination of bone erosions, cartilage degradation, and joint space narrowing, in addition to osteophyte formation, capsular ossification, and heterotopic calcification. Together with the characteristic joint distribution, this combination of radiographic features helps distinguish patients with SpA and psoriatic arthritis from those with RA. Secondary processes such as degenerative osteoarthritis and muscle weakness due to damage and disuse also contribute to pain and disability as the disease progresses.

While synthetic disease modifying anti-rheumatic drugs (sDMARDs) are considered to be ineffective for spinal and sacroiliac disease in axSpA, they have been used for peripheral joint involvement in axSpA. A Cochrane review of methotrexate treatment in AS did not report significant benefits for any outcomes, although a few individual studies suggested a non-significant reduction in number of swollen joints (Chen, 2013). Similarly, the Cochrane review of sulfasalazine in AS did not identify any clinically meaningful benefit (Chen, 2014). While in clinical practice sulfasalazine may be tried for peripheral joint involvement in clinical practice, most axSpA patients with significant disease will ultimately require treatment with TNF inhibitors, which have been shown to be effective for peripheral arthritis in axSpA.

Hips

Hip involvement in axSpA is generally a bad prognostic feature and can have a devastating effect on patients' function and quality of life. The prevalence of hip joint involvement in AS is reported to be between 20% and 35%, with hip involvement associated with a significantly worse Bath Ankylosing Spondylitis Functional Index (BASFI) compared to those with no hip involvement (Vander Cruyssen, 2010). Symptoms of hip involvement may also be incorrectly attributed to pain referred from the sacroiliac joints or lumbar spine and therefore overlooked. Therefore, hips should always be carefully examined in the clinic and actively inspected on the pelvic x-rays done to image the sacroiliac joints. Typical features on conventional radiographs include global, concentric joint space narrowing (as opposed to the more superior involvement in degenerative arthritis), erosions in the acetabulum, and osteoproliferation with osteophyte formation and capsular calcification. Rarely, complete ossification of the joint can occur. An example of severe hip disease in a patient with AS is shown in Figure 7.1.

Inflammation of the hip (coxofemoral) joints can begin at a young age. In one study in patients with juvenile SpA, hip joint osteitis was visualized on MRI in 45% of the children with a mean age of 12. Generally, the earlier a

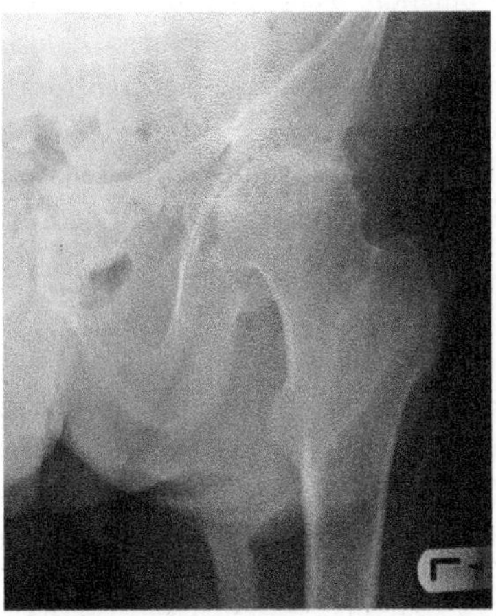

Fig. 7.1 Plain x-ray of the left hip in a patient with advanced ankylosing spondylitis demonstrating marked, and almost total, concentric joint space narrowing.

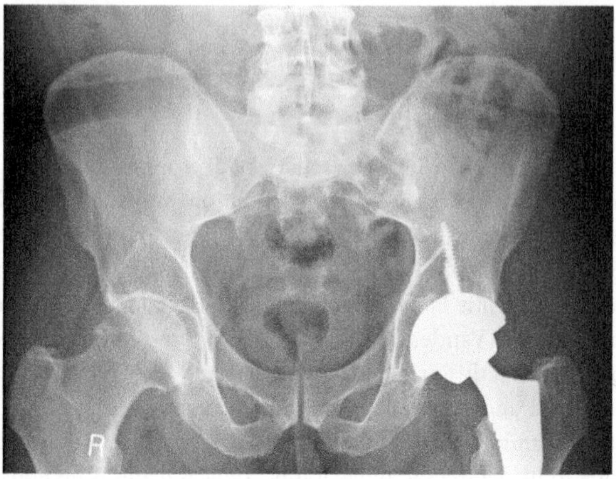

Fig. 7.2 Left total hip prosthesis in a patient with advanced ankylosing spondylitis. Evidence of right hip disease and sacroiliitis can also be seen.

patient develops hip involvement, the more severe the hip disease will be in adulthood. In addition, there is a strong association between severity of hip disease and the severity of axial spine disease, although age of onset and disease duration seems to be more influential for hip disease than axial disease.

The hip joints support most of the body's weight and are key in mobility, particularly ambulation. Patients with hip involvement often have higher pain and disability scores, and as such, the use of TNF inhibitors may be more commonly required in treatment. Historically, about 5–10% of patients required hip replacement surgery (see Figure 7.2), with half of these requiring bilateral replacements (Vander Cruyssen, 2010). The rate of hip joint replacement has likely decreased in the last decade with more effective treatments.

Knees

Patients with AS rarely present with synovitis of the knees, although this appears to be more common in axSpA. However, when patients do have significant knee effusions, these are often large and may recur fairly rapidly after aspiration and injection. Synovial biopsies from patients with AS showed less pannus formation, but more angiogenesis of the synovial membrane and more subchondral bone oedema, compared to patients with RA. Involvement of the tibiofibular joint of may also be seen more frequently in AS than RA.

Shoulders

With the shoulder being another 'root joint', patients with AS often have shoulder symptoms, with an estimated prevalence of 30%. Common sources of shoulder pain in AS include acromioclavicular joint (osteitis), supraspinatus tendonitis/enthesitis, joint capsulitis, and, less frequently, glenohumeral joint synovitis. In one study, 30% of AS patients had radiological changes, all of which were minor (Will, 2000). While shoulder involvement is relatively common, it generally does not lead to major disability or require joint replacement.

Temporomandibular joints

The temporomandibular joints (TMJs) have been reported to be more frequently involved in patients with AS than RA and health controls. Symptoms of TMJ involvement include headaches and painful jaw movements when eating or speaking. TMJ involvement may result in a variable range of motion of the joint, with some less mobile and some hypermobile, although presenting symptoms are generally similar (Ramos-Remus, 1997). Imaging findings include condylar and temporal erosions, sclerosis, TMJ articular disc displacement, and osseous degenerative changes.

Chest wall

Anterior chest wall pain affects approximately 45% of patients with axSpA. Costovertebral, manubriosternal, sternoclavicular, and costochondral joints can be involved, with the majority having involvement of more than one site. Both synovitis of the joints and enthesitis of joint capsules tend to occur. Involvement of these joints can often be observed as an incidental finding on spinal MRI scans.

A recent study used ultrasound to detect chest wall involvement in patients with SpA and found an incidence of 36.5% compared to 14% in normal subjects (Verhoeven, 2015). Erosions of the sternoclavicular joints and ankylosis of the manubriosternal joints were seen, particularly among those with a longer disease duration, radiographic sacroiliitis, and inflammatory bowel disease. Chest wall involvement can lead to discomfort and pain (often with localized tenderness), and limit chest expansion and ultimately restrict breathing, although this is increasingly rarely seen since the introduction of the TNF inhibitors.

Enthesitis

The enthesis is the site of insertion of tendon or ligament into bone. It is a complex structure composed of fibrocartilage, collagen fibres, synovium, and bursae, and may contain distinct populations of cells involved in inflammation. Enthesitis, inflammation of the enthesis, is often considered to be relatively specific to SpA-related conditions. However, the entheses are involved with repetitive mechanical loading, so transient enthesitis may also be a response to biomechanical stress in healthy individuals. Enthesitis has been reported to occur in 40–70% of patients at some point in their disease course, with the wide variation reflecting whether this is defined clinically or radiologically.

Clinically, patients with enthesitis may report pain and stiffness, occasionally with associated localized swelling, at entheseal sites (see Figure 7.3). This is often most apparent, and troublesome, in the Achilles tendon. Inflammatory enthesitis of the Achilles tendon is localized to the insertion of the tendon into the heel, and should be distinguished from the more common degenerative Achilles tendinopathy that affects the tendon more proximally, before it reaches the heel. This distinction can often be difficult clinically, in which case ultrasound or MRI imaging may be helpful. The Achilles and plantar fascia insertions into the calcaneus are the most commonly affected entheseal sites in axSpA and may have a major impact on a patient's mobility. Patients with axSpA who report heel pain should,

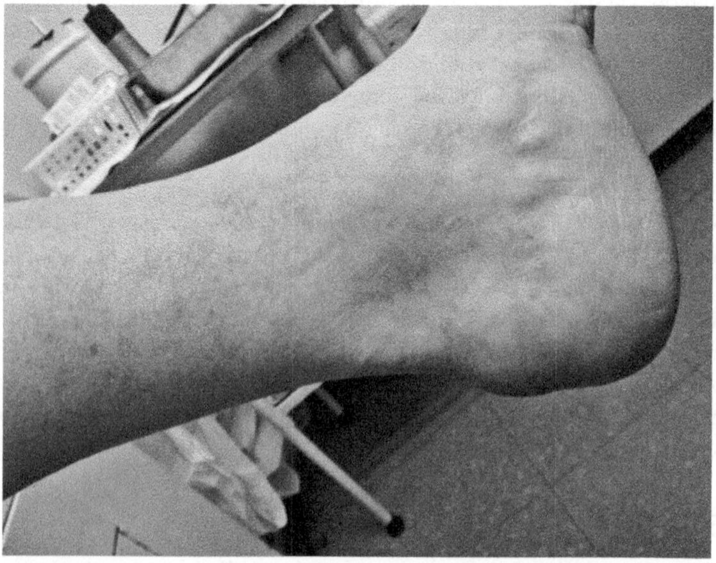

Fig. 7.3 Enthesitis of the Achilles tendon, with visible swelling at the entheseal insertion.

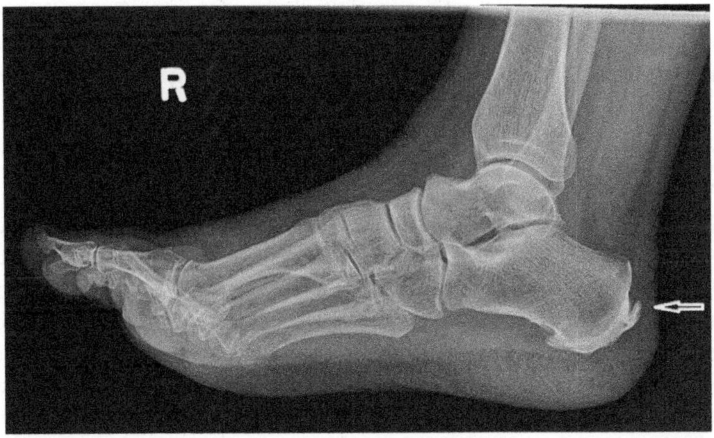

Fig. 7.4 Enthesiophyte formation (spur) at the Achilles enthesis (white arrow) and plantar fascia insertion in a patient with ankylosing spondylitis.

therefore, be evaluated for possible enthesitis at these sites. Calcaneal spurs are common x-ray findings in patients with axSpA (see Figure 7.4), but are not specific and are frequently also detected as incidental x-ray findings in those without disease.

Enthesitis can also occur at a large number of other sites including the patellar and quadriceps tendon insertions, greater trochanters, iliac crests, humeral tuberosity, elbow epicondyles, occiput, spinous processes, and costochondral joints. Tenderness of the entheseal point on clinical examination is usually used to detect enthesitis, although this is relatively insensitive and non-specific. Furthermore, many entheseal sites also overlap with tender points in fibromyalgia, so it can occasionally be difficult to distinguish these. Ultrasound and/or MRI are more sensitive than clinical examination, but less available and more expensive, so are usually reserved for when there is uncertainty with implications for treatment decisions.

Several scoring systems have been developed to objectify entheseal involvement in patients with axSpA, but these are time consuming and currently largely restricted to use in clinical trials. The scoring systems are covered in more detail in Chapter 13.

No randomized clinical trials in AS or axSpA have to date included enthesitis as primary outcome. One open-label study reported that adalimumab improved enthesitis in patients with active AS (Rudwaleit, 2010). In clinical practice, the other TNF inhibitors also appear effective for enthesitis, while the role of the IL-23 and IL-17 inhibitors should become clearer over the next few years. Further supporting evidence for the efficacy of these biologics for enthesitis, albeit as secondary outcome measure, is available from studies in the related condition of psoriatic arthritis.

Dactylitis

Dactylitis, or sausage digit, is a characteristic finding in both axial and peripheral SpA, as well as psoriatic arthritis. However, it is not specific and occasionally seen in a range of other rheumatic disorders. Therefore, context is important in attributing this to axSpA. Dactylitis is more commonly seen in axSpA patients with a personal or family history of psoriasis. Patients present with swelling of one or more digits, and while it is often painful and stiff in the early phase, it can also be relatively non-tender, particularly when it has been present for longer.

As opposed to the localized joint swelling seen with joint synovitis, dactylitis involves swelling of the entire digit. Dactylitis was traditionally thought to arise from the flexor tendons, with associated adjacent soft tissue swelling. However, recent high-resolution MRI analyses has indicated inflammation of entheseal sites, including the finger pulleys, fibrous sheaths, extensor tendons, as well as synovitis and osteitis, in addition to inflammation of the tendon sheaths.

Dactylitis has not been evaluated in any clinical trials in axSpA. Data from studies in psoriatic arthritis suggest TNF inhibitors may be helpful. It is, however, very uncommon for patients with axSpA to require treatment specifically for dactylitis, as they usually also have other, more symptomatic disease involvement requiring treatment.

Summary

While only present in a proportion of people with axSpA, peripheral musculoskeletal involvement is an important component of the disease with significant impact on function and quality of life. Many of the features may also be subtle and overlooked, unless specifically evaluated and examined. In particular, hip disease should be actively considered and, if present, may require more aggressive therapy or surgical intervention. On occasion, further imaging may be required to detect enthesitis or subtle joint inflammation in order to inform treatment decisions.

Key References and further reading

Chen J, Veras MM, Liu C, *et al.* Methotrexate for ankylosing spondylitis. *Cochrane Database Syst Rev.* 2013;2:CD004524. doi: 10.1002/14651858.CD004524.pub4.

Chen J, Lin S, Liu C. Sulfasalazine for ankylosing spondylitis. *Cochrane Database Syst Rev.* 2014;**11**:CD004800. doi: 10.1002/14651858.CD004800.pub3.

Dougados M, d'Agostino MA, Benessiano J, *et al.* The DESIR cohort: a 10-year follow-up of early inflammatory back pain in France: study design and baseline characteristics of the 708 recruited patients. *Joint Bone Spine.* 2011;**78**(6):598–603. doi: 10.1016/j.jbspin.2011.01.013.

Moltó A, Etcheto A, van der Heijde D, *et al.* Prevalence of comorbidities and evaluation of their screening in spondyloarthritis: results of the international cross-sectional ASAS-COMOSPA study. *Ann Rheum Dis.* 2016; 75(6):1016–23 doi: 10.1136/annrheumdis-2015-208174.

Ramos-Remus C, Major P, Gomez-Vargas A, *et al.* Temporomandibular joint osseous morphology in a consecutive sample of ankylosing spondylitis patients. *Ann Rheum Dis* 1997;**56**(2):103–7. doi:10.1136/ard.56.2.103

Rudwaleit M, Haibel H, Baraliakos X, *et al.* The early disease stage in axial spondyloarthritis: results from the German Spondyloarthritis Inception Cohort. *Arthritis Rheum.* 2009;**60**(3):717–27. doi: 10.1002/art.24483.

Rudwaleit M, Claudepierre P, Kron M, *et al.* Effectiveness of adalimumab in treating patients with ankylosing spondylitis associated with enthesitis and peripheral arthritis. *Arthritis Res Ther.* 2010;**12**(2):R43. doi: 10.1186/ar2953.

Will R, Kennedy G, Elswood J, *et al.* Ankylosing spondylitis and the shoulder: commonly involved but infrequently disabling. *J Rheumatol.* 2000;**27**(1):177–82. PMID: 10648036

Vander Cruyssen B, Muñoz-Gomariz E, Font P, *et al.* Hip involvement in ankylosing spondylitis: epidemiology and risk factors associated with hip replacement surgery. *Rheumatology* 2010;**49**(1):73–81. doi: 10.1093/rheumatology/kep174.

Vander Cruyssen B, Vastesaeger N, Collantes-Estevez E. Hip disease in ankylosing spondylitis. *Curr Opin Rheumatol.* 2013;**25**(4):448–54. doi: 10.1097/BOR.0b013e3283620e04.

Verhoeven F, Guillot X, Godfrin-Valnet M, *et al.* Ultrasonographic evaluation of the anterior chest wall in spondyloarthritis: a prospective and controlled study. *J Rheumatol.* 2015;**42**(1):87–92. doi: 10.3899/jrheum.

Chapter 8

Extra-articular manifestations of axial spondyloarthritis

Key points

- Axial spondyloarthritis (axSpA) is associated with a number of extra-articular manifestations (EAMs) reflecting shared clinical, genetic, and pathophysiological features.
- The EAMs are considered part of the spondyloarthritis spectrum and should be differentiated from complications arising as a consequence of the disease.
- The key EAMs of axSpA are inflammatory bowel disease (IBD), uveitis, and psoriasis.
- EAMs carry their own morbidity and often warrant treatment in their own right. Furthermore, the presence of EAMs may influence the choice of therapy used to treat the underlying axSpA.
- Clinicians should ensure that the EAMs of axSpA are actively and regularly enquired about when reviewing patients with axSpA.

Although axial spondyloarthritis (axSpA) is primarily considered a disease of the axial skeleton, several other organ systems can be affected, including peripheral joints, the skin, gastrointestinal tract, cardiovascular system, and eyes. The peripheral musculoskeletal features are covered in Chapter 7.

Over recent years, there has been an increased recognition of the importance of identifying and managing comorbidities in patients with chronic rheumatic conditions. Rheumatologists are advised to screen their patients for comorbidities and complications related to the rheumatic disease and treatments. The focus in rheumatoid arthritis (RA) has largely been on managing cardiovascular risk associated with this systemic condition. In contrast, in axSpA the emphasis is more on detecting and managing extra-articular manifestations (EAMs). EAMs should be differentiated from complications of axSpA; the EAMs are considered part of the spondyloarthritis

(SpA) spectrum, while the complications are generally a consequence of having the disease. The complications, which include musculoskeletal (osteoporosis, spinal fractures), cardiovascular, pulmonary, and renal involvement, are covered in Chapter 9. An overview of the key EAMs is shown in Figure 8.1.

The EAMs cluster together across the SpA family of disorders, reflecting their shared genetic and pathophysiological factors (covered in Chapters 4 and 5, respectively). Despite the high frequency and strength of these associations, causality cannot be assumed, and the relationship between the various manifestations is likely to be complex, involving a number of shared and unique processes.

As the EAMs often pre-date the diagnosis of axSpA, early identification and recognition of these associations can facilitate earlier diagnosis of axSpA. In fact, the Assessment of SpondyloArthritis international Society (ASAS) classification criteria for axSpA rely heavily on the presence or absence of EAMs, particularly in those patients without definite radiographic findings. In patients with an established diagnosis of axSpA, the identification

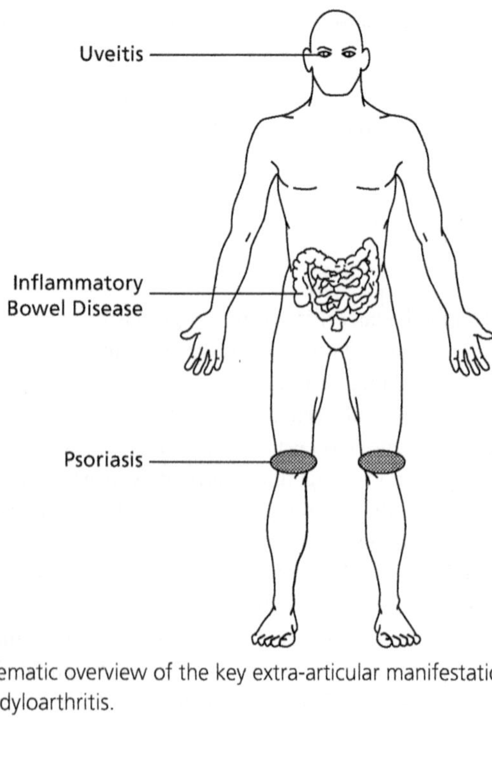

Fig. 8.1 Schematic overview of the key extra-articular manifestations (EAMs) in axial spondyloarthritis.

of EAMs is also important to guide overall treatment decisions, including selection of TNF inhibitor. The presence of co-morbid EAMs has been shown to be associated with worse prognosis, reduced quality of life, and worse work outcomes, compared to patients without EAMs. Patients with axSpA and significant gastrointestinal, skin or eye EAMs require multidisciplinary management, including a shared care model incorporating the relevant specialists. Several large academic centres deliver this in specific shared clinics between rheumatologists and gastroenterologists, dermatologists or ophthalmologists.

Inflammatory bowel disease (IBD)

Abdominal symptoms such as pain, diarrhoea, and bloating are common in patients with ankylosing spondylitis (AS). In a systematic review looking at EAMs in patients with AS, the pooled prevalence of IBD was 6.8%, although other studies have reported this to be as high as 15% (Stolwijk, 2015). An example of endoscopic features in IBD is shown in Figure 8.2. Furthermore, during endoscopy, mucosal ulcerations of the ileum and colon suggestive of subclinical IBD are seen macroscopically in 25–40% and microscopically in up to 60% of patients with AS (Mielants, 1995). In another SpA cohort, ileocolonoscopy revealed microscopic gut inflammation in approximately 50%, with acute and chronic lesions in 20% and 30%, respectively (Van Praet, 2013). About 20% of those patients with chronic lesions developed

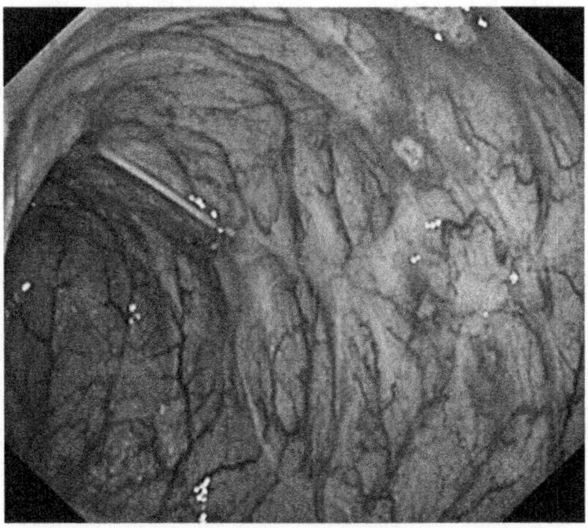

Fig. 8.2 Endoscopic image of the ileum in a patient with Crohn's disease. Several mucosal ulcerations and strictures are visible.

overt IBD over a 5-year period, suggesting chronic microscopic lesions may be an early form of IBD. Male sex, younger age, higher disease activity, and progressive disease were found to be independently associated with microscopic gut inflammation in patients with axSpA. No association was found for HLA-B27, non-steroidal anti-inflammatory drug (NSAID) use, or co-existence of other EAMs. Interestingly, resolution of intestinal inflammation often leads to resolution of joint and spinal pain, thus making it an important target for treatment considerations.

If the association is considered from the aspect of IBD, then approximately 5–10% of patients diagnosed with known IBD will develop confirmed AS. However, about 30% of patients with IBD have asymptomatic radiographic changes in the sacroiliac joints (often noted on CT scans done for abdominal symptoms), so the rates of non-radiographic axSpA (nr-axSpA) may be even higher.

While the association between joint and gut inflammation is well recognized in clinical practice and has been confirmed in several studies, the exact mechanism linking this association remains unclear. The mechanism is likely to relate to the shared genetic susceptibility factors (see Chapter 4), anomalous antigen processing in the gut, and subsequent IL-23/IL-17 pathway activation (see Chapter 5).

Therefore, patients with axSpA should be asked to report any gastrointestinal symptoms, with a low threshold for referral to a gastroenterologist for endoscopy if they have suggestive symptoms. NSAIDs have been reported to cause mucosal lesions and/or exacerbate IBD; however, this remains controversial due to limited study designs. One study using a COX-2 selective NSAID, celecoxib, did not show worsening of Crohn's disease. Given the beneficial effect of NSAIDs in the treatment of axSpA, it is recommended to discuss the option of ongoing use of NSAIDs in patients with axSpA and associated IBD with the patient's gastroenterology specialist as part of the shared care required for these patients. In these settings, it may be preferable to use COX-2 selective NSAIDs at low doses and for shorter periods of time.

Treatment for IBD may initially include oral corticosteroids, and immunomodulators such as sulfasalazine, mercaptopurine, 5-aminosalicylic acid, and methotrexate. While some of these may help the peripheral joints in axSpA, they are unlikely to benefit the axial symptoms. Several monoclonal antibody TNF inhibitors have been approved for use in patients with Crohn's disease, so these are often the preferred choice where there is ongoing active IBD and/or axSpA despite first line therapies. There are, however, several important differences between TNF inhibitors in IBD and axSpA that need to be considered when treating patients where these conditions co-exist. Firstly, while the soluble receptor protein etanercept has been shown to be effective in AS and nr-axSpA, etanercept is not effective as a treatment for Crohn's disease. Therefore, patients with active axSpA with confirmed or suspected IBD should be treated with a TNF monoclonal antibody, and not etanercept. Secondly, the treatment induction doses used for IBD are typically higher than those used in axSpA, so doses may occasionally need to be adjusted for these patients, in conjunction with their gastroenterologist. A meta-analysis of trials of AS patients on TNF inhibitors reported that new onset of IBD is an infrequent event in these patients, with no significant difference from placebo. However, in those with a previous history of IBD, there were significant differences between TNF inhibitors in terms of IBD flares. While infliximab was protective, etanercept use was associated with significantly increased odds of having an IBD flare. The role and safety of IL-23 and IL-17 inhibition in patients with axSpA and IBD still remains to be determined.

Uveitis

Acute anterior uveitis (AAU) is the most common EAM in AS, occurring in 25–35% of patients. AAU is characterized by intraocular inflammation of the iris, ciliary bodies, and/or choroids. Neutrophil infiltration and high levels of TNFα in the anterior chamber and uveal tract are implicated in the pathogenesis, but the underlying causation is still not fully understood. About 50% of all patients with AAU and 90% of AS patients with AAU are HLA-B27 positive. In cases of AAU without AS, other features of SpA, such as enthesitis, are more frequently detected by ultrasound than in patients without AAU, leading some authors to propose that isolated AAU may be an incomplete form of SpA. Uveitis forms an important component of the ASAS classification criteria. Therefore, patients presenting with inflammatory back pain or other features suggestive of SpA should always be asked specifically about this as they may have forgotten about previous episodes and not volunteer this information spontaneously.

Typically, patients with AAU present with a 1–2 day prodrome of mild unilateral eye discomfort followed by acute pain, redness, decreased acuity, and photophobia. Figure 8.3 demonstrates a typical example of AAU. Attacks can last for up to 6–12 weeks untreated, and commonly recur in either eye, with relapses more commonly seen in those who are HLA-B27 positive and those with longer AS disease duration. Males may manifest AAU more often than females. Ten percent of cases become chronic and can lead to permanent visual impairment if there is extension into the posterior chamber. In addition, if untreated patients may develop synechiae (adhesions), leading to pupil distortion, glaucoma, and cataracts. If AAU is suspected in a patient

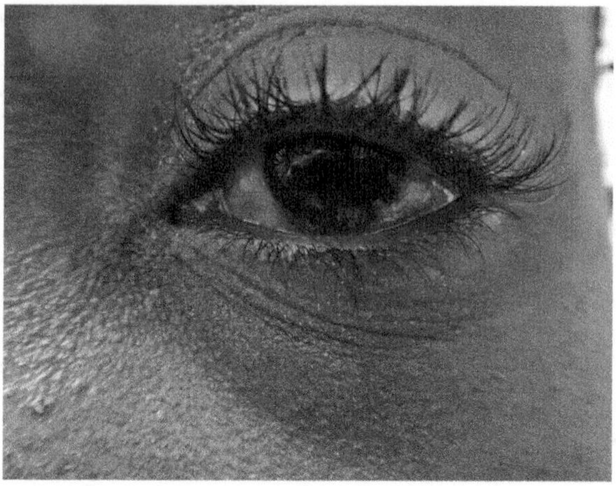

Fig. 8.3 Acute anterior uveitis affecting the left eye of a patient with ankylosing spondylitis.

with axSpA, then urgent referral to an ophthalmologist is recommended for definitive slit lamp examination and treatment to prevent complications.

The treatment of AAU is complex and should be done by a specialist ophthalmologist. Fortunately, the majority of patients are responsive to treatment and have a good prognosis. Initial therapies include topical glucocorticoids, to decrease anterior chamber inflammation, and dilating eye drops, to decrease pain from ciliary muscle spasm and to prevent posterior synechiae formation. If the AAU is resistant to topical treatments, then brief courses (usually 2 weeks) of oral corticosteroids, such as prednisone, or periocular corticosteroid injections can be used. Systemic treatment with methotrexate or rarely a TNF inhibitor may be required for some patients.

In patients with recurrent or frequent severe episodes of AAU, preventative strategies may be indicated. Sulfasalazine and, to a lesser extent, methotrexate have been shown to decrease the severity and frequency of AAU flares, while oral NSAIDs may also have some preventative effects. More recently, TNF inhibitors have been shown to be effective in reducing flares of AAU in patients with AS. In a large open label trial of adalimumab in AS patients, the overall flare rate was reduced by 50%. A variety of TNF inhibitors have been shown to be effective in decreasing flares of AAU in AS patients, with some evidence to suggest that etanercept may be less effective than the monoclonal anti-TNF antibodies (namely infliximab and adalimumab), although this remains somewhat controversial and may relate to methodological issues relating to reporting.

Interestingly, TNF inhibitors have also been reported to occasionally cause AAU, with etanercept the most commonly reported agent. However, it is difficult to attribute causality to a treatment in patients with a condition like AS where AAU is part of the disease spectrum. Reassuringly, uveitis is rarely reported in RA where TNF inhibitors are widely used.

Psoriasis

Psoriasis is a chronic, inflammatory skin disease which affects approximately 2% of the Caucasian population. Plaque psoriasis is the most common form, and is characterized by raised, erythematous and scaly lesions, often on the scalp and extensor surfaces (see Figure 8.4). In patients with AS, psoriasis is present in approximately 10%, varying geographically, with the highest rates in Europe (11%) and lowest in East Asia (3%).

In a large AS cohort, patients with concomitant psoriasis had a worse disease course and more frequent peripheral joint involvement compared to AS patients without psoriasis. While the HLA-B27 allele does not seem pathogenetically implicated in the development of plaque psoriasis, patients that are HLA-B27 positive usually have an onset of psoriasis at a later age (50–60 years).

While psoriasis can often be treated effectively with topical measures, in patients with more troublesome psoriasis, referral to a dermatologist is suggested. In these cases, measures such as UV phototherapy, acitretin,

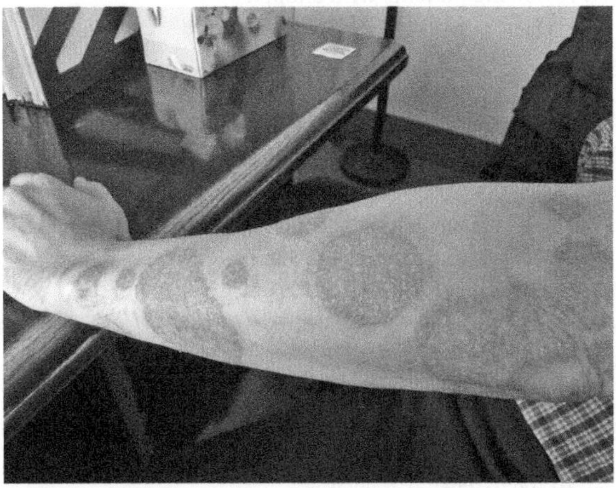

Fig. 8.4. Extensive plaque psoriasis affecting the extensor surfaces of a patient's arm.

cyclosporine, and methotrexate are often effective. While most of these measures are effective for the skin, they generally do not improve the underlying axial disease. In contrast, TNF inhibitors are effective for both refractory psoriasis and axSpA. There are also several newer agents, such as apremilast, ustekinumab, and secukinumab, available for the treatment of psoriasis and psoriatic arthritis, although studies investigating their efficacy in AS and axSpA are still ongoing. Similar to the case with uveitis, there are also case reports of TNF inhibitors paradoxically triggering various forms of psoriasis, which usually resolve upon discontinuation of the agent.

Summary

EAMs are an important component of axSpA and reinforce the SpA concept with shared clinical, genetic, and pathophysiological features. EAMs carry their own morbidity and often warrant treatment in their own right. Furthermore, the presence of EAMs, particularly IBD and AAU, may influence the choice of therapy used to treat the underlying axSpA. Decisions regarding which component of the disease should take priority for treatment depend on the severity of the individual components, but there are now therapies available that can effectively and simultaneously treat multiple SpA components. However, dichotomous responses in different tissue compartments remain common, so there remains unmet need in the treatment of patients with axSpA and significant EAMs. Clinicians should ensure that the well-recognized EAMs of axSpA are actively and regularly enquired about when reviewing patients with axSpA.

Key References and further reading

Elewaut D, Matucci-Cerinic M. Treatment of ankylosing spondylitis and extra-articular manifestations in everyday rheumatology practice. *Rheumatology (Oxford)*. 2009;**48**(9):1029–35. doi: 10.1093/rheumatology/kep146.

Jacques P, Van Praet L, Carron P, *et al.* Pathophysiology and role of the gastrointestinal system in spondyloarthritides. *Rheum Dis Clin North Am*. 2012;**38**(3):569–82. doi: 10.1016/j.rdc.2012.08.012.

Mielants H, Veys EM, Cuvelier C, *et al.* The evolution of spondyloarthropathies in relation to gut histology. II. Histological aspects. *J Rheumatol*. 1995;**22**(12):2273–8. PMID: 8835561

Rosenbaum JT. Uveitis in spondyloarthritis including psoriatic arthritis, ankylosing spondylitis, and inflammatory bowel disease. *Clin Rheumatol*. 2015;**34**(6):999–1002. doi: 10.1007/s10067-015-2960-8.

Stolwijk C, van Tubergen A, Castillo-Ortiz JD, *et al.* Prevalence of extra-articular manifestations in patients with ankylosing spondylitis: a systematic review and meta-analysis. *Ann Rheum Dis.* 2015;**74**(1):65–73. doi: 10.1136/annrheumdis-2013-203582.

Van Praet L, Van den Bosch FE, Jacques P, *et al.* Microscopic gut inflammation in axial spondyloarthritis: a multiparametric predictive model. *Ann Rheum Dis.* 2013;**72**(3):414–17. doi: 10.1136/annrheumdis-2012-202135.

Zeboulon N, Dougados M, Gossec L. Prevalence and characteristics of uveitis in the spondyloarthropathies: a systematic literature review. *Ann Rheum Dis.* 2008;**67**(7):955–59. doi:10.1136/ard.2007.075754.

Chapter 9

Complications of axial spondyloarthritis

Key points

- In addition to the well-recognized extra-articular manifestations (EAMs) of ankylosing spondylitis (AS), this condition can also be associated with a number of clinically important complications.
- Patients with AS are at increased risk of osteoporosis and spinal fractures. The latter may occur after seemingly minor trauma and may lead to significant neurological compromise.
- Other potential neurological complications include atlantoaxial subluxation and compressive radiculopathy or myelopathy.
- Cardiac complications include cardiovascular events, valvular disease, and conduction disturbances.
- Pulmonary disease in AS relates to parenchymal involvement or mechanical constraint from chest wall inflammation.
- Renal disease is generally rare in AS.

In addition to the well-recognized extra-articular manifestations (EAMs; covered in Chapter 8) of axial spondyloarthritis (axSpA), this condition can also be associated with a number of clinically important complications. While the EAMs are considered part of the spondyloarthritis (SpA) spectrum, the complications are generally a consequence of having the disease. Most of the literature published about complications pre-dates the Assessment of SpondyloArthritis international Society (ASAS) criteria for axSpA, and therefore relates to ankylosing spondylitis (AS) rather that the broader definition of axSpA. An overview of the key complications in AS is shown in Figure 9.1.

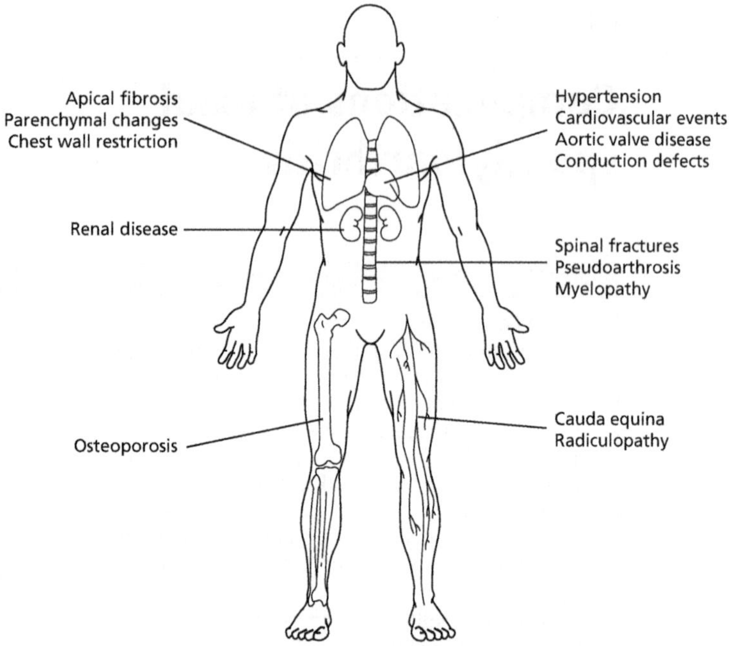

Fig. 9.1 Schematic overview of the key complications in axial spondyloarthritis.

Osteoporosis

Reduced bone mineral density (BMD) is a common complication, occurring in over 60% of patients with AS. Osteoporosis affects approximately 20% of patients, and has been linked to the development of vertebral fractures. While decreased BMD in the spine and hip is associated with increased disease duration, bone loss may also occur early in the course of the disease. A systematic review reported prevalence rates between 51–54% for low BMD and 13–16% for osteoporosis in patients with AS (predominantly male) within 10 years of diagnosis (van der Weijden, 2012).

Persistent spinal inflammation, as assessed by spinal stiffness and acute phase reactants, was associated with lower BMD. The pathogenesis of osteoporosis in AS patients is complex, involving local factors, such as TNFα, which increase bone mineral turnover, and altered mechanics leading to less weight bearing, shear stress, and subsequent bone loss.

In clinical practice, dual energy x-ray absorptiometry (DEXA) is commonly used to assess BMD. However, with advanced AS, particularly when there is superimposed periosteal bone and syndesmophyte formation, DEXA scanning can provide falsely elevated measurements. In one study, lateral lumbar DEXA (in which DEXA is done with the patient on their side) yielded significantly lower BMD and more cases of osteoporosis, compared with standard antero-posterior DEXA. Development of osteoporosis in that study correlated with age, disease duration, inflammatory markers, and low body mass index. Another study used high-resolution peripheral quantitative CT scans to assess bone quality and demonstrated that cortical parameters, such as thickness and porosity, were diminished as were bone stiffness and strength in the AS patients. These bone changes were also present in non-axial skeletal sites, such as the distal radius. Therefore some uncertainty remains how best to measure and interpret BMD in patients with axSpA.

Bisphosphonates are not traditionally used routinely to treat osteoporosis in AS patients as their effects on proliferative bone formation are uncertain. Treating disease-related inflammation, particularly with non-steroidal anti-inflammatory drugs (NSAIDs) and TNF inhibitors, has been shown to be an effective strategy in reversing bone loss, although one recent study indicated that new spinal fractures still occurred during 4 years of treatment with TNF inhibitors. Vitamin D supplementation, regular physiotherapy, and reducing other risk factors, such as alcohol and smoking, are also important treatment strategies in this population.

Spinal fractures and neurologic injury

Changes in the bony microarchitecture and biomechanics of the spine predispose AS patients to vertebral fractures following seemingly trivial trauma. The prevalence of vertebral fractures in patients with AS has been estimated to be between 4% and 18%, depending on disease duration. The lifetime risk of vertebral fractures in AS patients has been estimated to be four times higher than in unaffected persons. Most spinal fractures occur in the lower cervical spine, followed by the thoracic spine. A significant proportion may develop multilevel fractures. Spinal fractures in AS are typically horizontal and occur through the ossified disc (transdiscal) or the vertebral body (transcorporal) as a result of extension-distraction forces, usually hyperextension injuries. If there continues to be persistent motion at the fracture site, a pseudarthrosis may develop. This is seen as irregular osteolysis of the endplate, sclerosis, and vacuum phenomenon of the disc space.

Assessment and diagnosis of vertebral fractures may be difficult as patients already have longstanding spinal pain and may deny any significant injury. Therefore, a high clinical suspicion is required in patients with AS reporting even fairly minor trauma, particularly in those patients known to have multilevel ankylosis. In fact, any AS patients with new onset acute neck pain or sudden change in posture (regardless of whether or not this is painful)

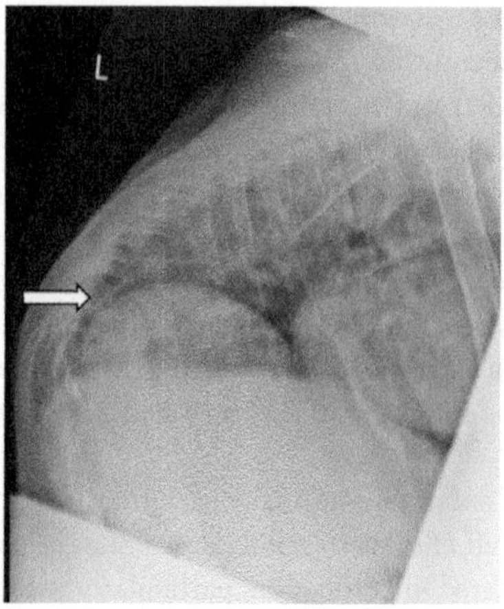

Fig. 9.2 X-ray of severe kyphotic deformity, with extensive fusion and suspicion of pseudoarthrosis (arrow) of the thoracic spine in a patient with advanced ankylosing spondylitis.

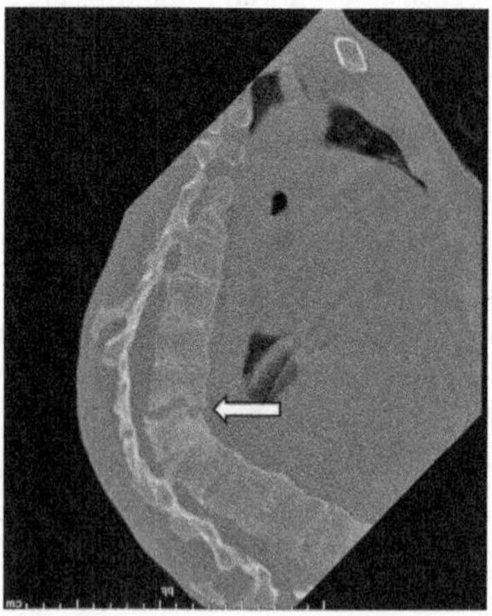

Fig. 9.3 CT scan of same patient as Figure 9.2 confirming pseudoarthrosis (arrow) of ankylosed spine.

should be assumed to have a fracture until proven otherwise. Furthermore, radiographic evaluation is complicated by the presence of existing changes due to the underlying AS, making it difficult to visualize fractures on plain films. If a spinal fracture is suspected but not seen on plain films, then further imaging with CT and/or MRI scans is indicated (see Figures 9.2 and 9.3

for x-ray and CT of spinal fracture). One study indicated that a significant number of fractures may be missed on just a single modality, suggesting that CT and MRI can be considered complementary modalities for detecting fractures in patients with AS where clinical suspicion is very high or in planning spinal surgery.

Not only are spinal fractures increased in AS, but the risk of associated spinal cord injury is significantly increased. Sixty-five percent of spinal fractures in AS are reported to be associated with some degree of neurological complication. Pre-existing multilevel bony ankylosed sections act like rigid long levers, making the fractures unstable and significantly increasing the risk of neurological compromise. While most patients present with no or only subtle neurologic symptoms following minor trauma, subsequent displacement can lead to paraparesis or quadriparesis.

The treatment of spinal fractures in AS differs considerably from the treatment of these fractures in the general population due to the altered biomechanics and inherent instability of the fractures. Immobilization and protected transfers are mandatory to reduce the risk of spinal cord compression. It is recommended that patients with ankylosed spines should carry a medical alert card notifying emergency responders to avoid unnecessary manipulation of the neck and to use caution if endotracheal intubation is required. While surgical treatment is usually required and recommended due to the instability of the fractures, non-surgical management has been used in certain circumstances in the past. However, the most common reasons for non-surgical management are generally due to unacceptably high surgical risk and patient refusal of surgical treatment. The management options for spinal fractures in AS were reviewed in a recent paper by Werner et al. (2016). Complication rates following nonsurgical or surgical management in AS are higher than those in the general population.

Other neurological complications

The majority of neurological manifestations in axSpA are related to spinal cord or radicular nerve compression due to fracture/dislocation, atlanto-axial subluxation, or compression as a result of new bone formation.

Spinal fractures have been covered in more detail earlier in this chapter. It should be noted that spinal fractures can lead to both acute onset and more slowly evolving neurological symptoms, so patients with fused spines and neurological symptoms should always be specifically asked about episodes of even seemingly trivial trauma.

Atlantoaxial subluxation (spinal level C1-C2) is another mechanism leading to spinal cord compression. Atlantoaxial subluxation may occur as a result of traumatic fracture-dislocation or pannus formation, although the latter is far less common than in rheumatoid arthritis (RA). While a minority present with just neck pain, two-thirds of patients have sensory disturbances, and a third have cranial neuropathy. Clinical signs include myelopathy, weakness, and decreased range of motion of the cervical spine. One study reported a prevalence of 14% for anterior atlantoaxial subluxation (>3mm) in 819 patients with AS. Of these, 32% had progressed after 2 years, by an average rate of 0.5 mm/year (Lee, 2012). Risk factors for progression included the presence of peripheral arthritis, elevated CRP, and active disease despite NSAIDs. In acute atlantoaxial subluxation, immediate management with immobilization and urgent surgical evaluation is required.

Rarely, cauda equina syndrome can present in patients with long-standing disease, often in those with significant spinal ankylosis. The lower lumbar and sacral nerves develop adhesions and fibrosis, likely due to chronic arachnoiditis, which can be manifest as dural ectasia on CT and MRI. Typically, saddle anesthesia, loss of bladder and bowel control, impotence, sensory loss, and/or weakness present in a subacute manner. Treatment is generally surgical.

Other rare neurological syndromes have been reported, including monophasic peripheral neuropathies and subclinical myopathies, although they are usually asymptomatic. Multiple-sclerosis (MS)-like white matter lesions can very rarely occur in AS patients treated with TNF inhibitors, as they do in other inflammatory diseases; the pathogenesis of these is likely to be related to the treatment rather than the underlying disease.

Cardiovascular complications

Rates of cardio- and cerebrovascular events, such as myocardial infarction and stroke, are known to be significantly higher in patients with chronic inflammatory conditions like RA than in the general population. While these rates also appear to be increased in patients with AS, compared to the general population, these are generally lower than those reported for RA. As with other rheumatic diseases, chronic inflammation may be a risk factor contributing to endothelial dysfunction, although systemic levels of inflammation are generally far lower in axSpA than RA, which may partly explain the differential rates of cardiovascular disease. Traditional cardiovascular risk factors are generally higher in patients with AS compared to the general population, while physical activity is often limited due to pain and reduced mobility leading to a more sedentary lifestyle. In addition, therapies such as NSAIDs may be pro-thrombotic and lead to increased cardiovascular events, although this remains controversial. In fact, there are some studies suggesting that NSAIDs may even have beneficial cardiac effects in patients with AS as they decrease the inflammatory state.

In a recent meta-analysis involving 27,532 patients with AS with a mean follow-up of 15 years, significant increases in myocardial infarction (odds ratio = 1.60) and stroke (odds ratio = 1.50) were estimated in AS patients compared to controls (Mathieu, 2015). However, other studies using population-based cohort data and carefully controlling for a variety of cardiovascular risk factors have reported far lower estimates, some of which do not differ significantly from the general population. Most of the studies have, however, reported an increased association of AS with hypertension. The mechanism for this is unclear, but may relate in part to the widespread use of NSAIDs in AS.

Therefore, the true risk for cardiovascular disease in AS remains unclear at this stage. While many guidelines include recommendations for screening for cardiovascular risk factors, the best strategy for this in clinical practice remains unclear. The current evidence supports regular monitoring of blood pressure and treatment of hypertension, while all patients who smoke should be actively encouraged and supported to quit.

Cardiac valve and conduction complications

Aortic root disease has been reported in patients with AS. Transoesophageal echocardiographic studies identified fibrosis of the aortic root and membranous interventricular septum in 61% of patients with AS. Thickened valvular leaflets lead to a characteristic 'sub-aortic bump' seen on echocardiography in about 30% of asymptomatic patients with AS. Aortic regurgitation, due to fibrotic thickening of the aortic valves, has been estimated to occur in 5–10% of patients with AS. Aortic regurgitation in AS rarely requires valve replacement, and no aortic aneurysm ruptures have been reported.

Conduction disturbances, most commonly P-R prolongation, due to fibrosis of the septum and nodes, are estimated to occur in 3–33%. HLA-B27 may be a contributing factor in conduction disturbances in patients with SpA, while severe conduction disturbances have also been reported in HLA-B27-positive patients without SpA. It is important to note that most of these studies were small, uncontrolled, and used different techniques in assessment. Overall, the conduction abnormalities were minor and rarely symptomatic.

In a cross-sectional study, 100 male patients with AS of at least 15 years' duration underwent electrocardiograms and echocardiograms (Brunner,

2006). While there was a trend towards an increased rate of aortic and mitral regurgitation, this was not statistical significant, and conduction disturbances were similar to the general population. An increased frequency of left ventricular diastolic dysfunction compared to the general population was noted in this study and others. Inflammatory infiltrates were not found in myocardial biopsies, suggesting this may be an effect of hypertension, which was higher in the AS population, rather than directly due to inflammation. Other cardiac manifestations rarely reported in AS include myocarditis and pericarditis. The current data do not support routine echocardiography in asymptomatic patients with AS.

Pulmonary complications

Pulmonary disease in AS relates to both parenchymal involvement and mechanical constraint from chest wall inflammation. Diminished chest wall expansion, particularly due to costochondral and costovertebral joint inflammation and ankylosis can lead to restrictive pulmonary disease. Entheseal involvement of the anterior chest wall can result in pleuritic pain and result in shallow breathing. Although about 20% of patients with AS have a mild restrictive pattern on pulmonary function tests, the large majority are not limited by this, and further intervention is rarely needed. Treating chest wall inflammation pharmacologically, as part of controlling overall disease activity, often improves the restriction.

Reports of parenchymal fibrobullous disease date back to the 1940s, when upper lung zone fibrosis was detected on chest x-rays in patients with AS. Studies looking at apical parenchymal changes on plain film reported prevalence rates of 1–25%. High-resolution CT studies report pulmonary involvement between 40% and 80%, with a mean prevalence of 61% in a systematic review of 10 studies (El Maghraoui, 2012). The main findings on CT are non-specific interstitial abnormalities in the majority, followed by apical fibrosis, ground-glass attenuation, emphysema, and bronchiectasis. Apical fibrosis was related to disease duration, although this may be present even in early AS. Pulmonary function testing demonstrated a restrictive pattern in 34% of patients. In other studies involving AS patients with apical changes on x-ray, bronchoalveolar lavage was usually normal, while transbronchial biopsies indicated interstitial fibrosis without alveolitis. Overall, parenchymal pulmonary involvement is largely asymptomatic and rarely requires specific treatment. However, the apical distribution on imaging may on occasion be suggestive of pulmonary tuberculosis, which may cause concern when the use of TNF inhibitors is being considered. Other, far less frequently reported pulmonary manifestations include spontaneous pneumothorax, obstructive sleep apnea, and bacterial superinfection in those on immunosuppressive therapy.

Renal disease

Renal disease is generally rare in AS patients and, as such, studies are limited to case reports and retrospective studies. The most reported renal manifestations are AA amyloidosis and IgA nephropathy. In a retrospective cohort of 681 patients with AS, abnormal urinalysis (proteinuria and/or hematuria) was noted in 8%, with renal biopsy conducted in six patients with proteinuria over 1 g daily (Lee, 2013). Of these, three patients had a non-specific glomerulonephropathy, two patients had IgA nephropathy, and one had amyloidosis. Another retrospective study, using administrative data of 8,616 patients with AS, reported an overall prevalence of renal complications in 3.4% of males and 2.1% of females in the AS group compared to 2.0% and 1.6% in the general population (Levy, 2014). However, NSAID use was not documented and may be a significant contributory factor in kidney disease. Renal amyloidosis was five-times higher in those aged ≥60 years, suggesting a longer disease duration is contributory, typically in the setting of a high inflammatory state.

Key References and further reading

Brunner F, Kunz A, Weber U, *et al.* Ankylosing spondylitis and heart abnormalities: do cardiac conduction disorders, valve regurgitation and diastolic dysfunction occur more often in male patients with diagnosed ankylosing spondylitis for over 15 years than in the normal population? *Clin Rheumatol.* 2006;**25**(1):24–9. doi: 10.1007/s10067-005-1117-6

El Maghraoui A, Dehhaoui M. Prevalence and characteristics of lung involvement on high resolution computed tomography in patients with ankylosing spondylitis: A systematic review. *Pulm Med.* 2012:965956. doi: 10.1155/2012/965956.

Lee JS, Lee S, Bang SY, *et al.* Prevalence and risk factors of anterior atlantoaxial subluxation in ankylosing spondylitis. *J Rheumatol.* 2012;**39**(12):2321–6. doi: 10.3899/jrheum.120260.

Lee SH, Lee EJ, Chung SW, *et al.* Renal involvement in ankylosing spondylitis: prevalence, pathology, response to TNF-a blocker. *Rheumatol Int.* 2013;**33**(7):1689–92. doi: 10.1007/s00296-012-2624-9.

Levy AR, Szabo SM, Rao SR, *et al.* Estimating the occurrence of renal complications among persons with ankylosing spondylitis. *Arthritis Care Res.* 2014;**66**(3):440–5. doi: 10.1002/acr.22176.

Mathieu S, Pereira B, Soubrier M. Cardiovascular events in ankylosing spondylitis: an updated meta-analysis. *Semin Arthritis Rheum.* 2015;**44**(5):551–555. doi: 10.1016/j.semarthrit.2014.10.007.

Merciea C, van der Horst-Bruinsma IE, Borg AA. Pulmonary, renal and neurological comorbidities in patients with ankylosing spondylitis; implications for clinical practice. *Curr Rheumatol Rep.* 2014;**16**(8):434. doi: 10.1007/s11926-014-0434-7.

van der Weijden MA, Claushuis TA, Nazari T, *et al.* High prevalence of low bone mineral density in patients within 10 years of onset of ankylosing spondylitis: a systematic review. *Clin Rheumatol.* 2012;**31**(11):1529–35. doi: 10.1007/s10067-012-2018-0.

Vinsonneau U, Brondex A, Mansourati J, *et al.* Cardiovascular disease in patients with spondyloarthropathies. *Joint Bone Spine* 2008;75(1):18–21. doi:10.1016/j.jbspin.2007.04.011.

Werner BC, Samartzis D, Shen FH. Spinal fractures in patients with ankylosing spondylitis: etiology, diagnosis, and management. *J Am Acad Orthop Surg.* 2016;**24**(4):241–9. doi: 10.5435/JAAOS-D-14-00149.

Chapter 10

The impact and cost of axial spondyloarthritis

Key points

- Patients with ankylosing spondylitis (AS) and axial spondyloarthritis (axSpA) consistently report lower health-related quality of life compared to the general population.
- The effects of the condition include factors such as pain, reduced mobility, poor sleep, fatigue, and depression, with a similar burden of disease in patients with non-radiographic axSpA and established AS.
- AxSpA also significantly impacts on social and work participation. Patients with AS have lower work participation and are more likely to retire earlier than the general population. Those patients in work have reduced work productivity, due to absenteeism (ability to attend work) and presenteeism (productivity while at work).
- The financial cost of AS varies significantly between countries.

Axial spondyloarthritis (axSpA) is a chronic condition with significant impact on many aspects of a patient's quality of life. Many of these effects are not adequately captured by healthcare professionals during clinical consultations, where the emphasis is largely on disease activity, function, and treatment. The effects of axSpA include direct physical and psychosocial factors such as pain, reduced mobility, poor sleep, fatigue, and depression. Pain and fatigue are frequently identified by patients as the most disabling aspects of their disease. In addition, axSpA also significantly impacts on social and work participation. While many of these factors are also reported in other chronic rheumatic conditions, the impact on social development and attainment are particularly marked in axSpA as disease onset is typically in the second or third decades of life, which are crucial times for social and career development.

Overall, a similar burden of disease has been demonstrated in patients with non-radiographic axSpA (nr-axSpA) and established ankylosing spondylitis (AS). The only significant differences are in functional and metrology indices, due to the effect of more structural damage in those with established AS. Disability and loss of function, including aspects such as loss of independence, emotional distress, and decreased social functioning tend to develop within the first 10 years after disease onset (Gran, 1997). Therefore, the well-documented delay in diagnosis impacts on the burden of disease, with worse disease outcomes, higher levels of depression, and difficulties with social participation. It is hoped that earlier recognition of the condition, with timely introduction of effective therapies, could lead to reduced long-term impact, although this remains to be formally proven.

Quality of life

Quality of life is considered an important parameter in any long-term condition. Patients with AS consistently report lower health-related quality of life compared to the general population. Recent studies have confirmed that the quality of life in axSpA, including early disease, is also reduced and comparable to that seen in established AS. The disease impacts both the physical and mental components that make up health-related quality of life. There is good evidence that effective control of disease activity with TNF inhibitors improves quality of life in axSpA. While this improvement is generally considered clinically significant, health-related quality of life does not return to 'normal' levels in most patients.

It should also be noted that comorbidities associated with axSpA, particularly inflammatory bowel disease and psoriasis, may confer significant additional detrimental effects on quality of life. A largely underreported but important aspect is the effect on patients' sexual life. While this aspect correlates with quality of life measures, a recent study indicated that most patients do not talk about this with their partners or with healthcare professionals.

Fatigue

Significant fatigue is reported in over 50% of patients with AS, compared to 15–25% of the general population. In a large cohort of patients with axSpA, the prevalence of severe fatigue was 67%, and similar in those with AS and nr-axSpA (Bedaiwi, 2015). Patients with axSpA consistently identify fatigue as one of the symptoms with the largest negative impact on their quality of life. Fatigue is one of the components of the Bath Ankylosing Spondyloarthritis

Disease Activity Index (BASDAI), and therefore influences measures of disease activity and treatment decisions (see Chapters 13 and 15).

The association of fatigue and axSpA is complex and poorly understood. In axSpA, fatigue does not relate directly to depression, anxiety, or motivation, but has been suggested to relate mainly to pain (Brophy, 2013). Sleep problems are also an underreported issue in axSpA, as they are not captured by most of the standard outcome measures used in axSpA (covered in Chapter 13). While disease activity measures and inflammatory markers positively correlate with fatigue scores, fatigue does not always improve with treatment. Other associations with fatigue include female gender, inflammatory low back pain, hip involvement, enthesitis, peripheral arthritis, and sedentary lifestyle. In some patients, fatigue may also be part of associated fibromyalgia or an adverse effect of medications.

The treatment of fatigue can be difficult and remains an area of significant unmet need in axSpA. While TNF inhibitors improve disease activity and reduce inflammation in most patients, the effects on fatigue are often more limited, with fatigue remaining unresponsive or troublesome in a large proportion of patients. It is hoped that non-pharmacological strategies, such as cognitive behavioral therapy or mindfulness-based stress reduction, which are currently being evaluated in a number of studies, may prove beneficial for pain and fatigue in axSpA.

Work participation and productivity

Over the past decade there has been an increased recognition that AS and, more recently also axSpA, are associated with significant risk of reduced work participation and productivity. With the introduction of high-cost treatments for axSpA and other chronic rheumatic conditions, there has been great interest in defining the impact of the disease and these expensive therapies on work productivity (the key measures used to assess the effect of disease on work are covered in Chapter 13).

Withdrawal from work is three times more common in people with AS than in the general population. A recent UK cohort study indicated that ~40% of adults with AS were not working and that people with AS retired on average 9.5 years earlier than the general population (Cooksey, 2015).

Of those patients currently in work, productivity at work is reduced, as is the ability to perform household activities. Importantly, AS impacts on both the ability to attend work (absenteeism) and productivity while at work (presenteeism). While the former may be captured and noted by employers, the latter is often largely 'hidden'. A number of studies have reported that 14–50% of people with AS in paid employment had taken sick leave over a period of 2 years. There are significant country and cultural differences, which accounts for the wide range. In countries, such as the USA, where sick leave was low, a third of patients reported that they had needed to reduce working hours due to their AS. Productivity loss while at work (presenteeism) has been estimated to be around 21–30% for patients with AS. Presenteeism is therefore the major contributor to overall work impairment in AS, estimated to contribute between 26–53%, with the range again reflecting differences in absenteeism rates between countries.

The reasons for in-work disability are varied and include direct physical effects (pain, stiffness and reduced mobility), fatigue, impaired concentration and psychological factors linked to the condition. Work disability has been shown to be significantly associated with high disease activity (BASDAI) and functional impairment (BASFI), with the prevalence of work disability increasing with disease duration. Therefore, strategies to reduce work disability are expected to have the highest impact early in the disease and before patients lose their jobs. Work-related contextual factors, such as the number of hours worked, type of work, workplace and job satisfaction also contribute to work limitation in these patients (Boonen, 2015). This suggests that strategies to improve work should address both health-related and work-related factors.

It should also be noted that many studies have not evaluated impairment in unpaid work or activity. Patients who are not in paid employment are more likely to be older, and have longer disease duration and higher disease severity. Mean disease activity and, more importantly, functional impairment (BASFI), are higher in people with AS who are not working compared to those in paid employment. One study reported that overall activity impairment due to ill-health was 33% for those in work (work and home) and 52% for those not in work (home) (Cooksey, 2015). People not in work also report an increased need for formal and informal (friends and family) support or care. Therefore, much of the work and activity impairment associated with axSpA is 'hidden' and cannot be accurately calculated just from work participation rates.

Financial cost

AxSpA has significant economic effects on the individual patient, their family, healthcare funders, and society as a whole. Quantifying the true cost of AS is complex and estimates vary significantly between countries, mainly as a result of how healthcare is funded and whether patients are eligible for compensation or benefit payments. While estimates of the total cost of AS vary greatly, studies have consistently indicated that the majority of the costs of the condition are due to work-related factors, particularly early retirement and inefficient working (presenteeism). The direct healthcare costs are a smaller component, although with the introduction of the TNF inhibitors and Assessment of SpondyloArthritis international Society imaging criteria, the distribution of these costs has shifted from physiotherapy to drug and imaging-related costs. In addition, patients with AS also have significant out-of-pocket costs associated with their disease.

The key predictors of increased cost in the early years of disease are functional impairment and high disease activity, while lower quality of life predicts increased cost later in the disease (Palla, 2012). Country, age, and gender also have a significant impact on costs. There is significant variation in how studies have captured items or activities and attributed costs. Therefore, it is not easy to compare results across studies, particularly where these were performed in different countries. In the UK, a patient questionnaire study estimated the mean annual cost associated with AS to be £11,207 (Rafia, 2012). A more recent UK study, using a combination of linked routine and patient-reported data, estimated the mean total cost of AS to be £19,016 (95%CI: 14,854–23,149) per person per year (Cooksey, 2015). In their assessment of TNF inhibitor use for the treatment of AS and nr-axSpA, the National Institute for Health and Care Excellence (NICE) concluded that the use of these agents can be considered a cost-effective use of NHS resources. This treatment is likely to become more cost-effective in future with the introduction of less expensive biosimilar agents and resultant downward pressure on the cost of the existing innovator drugs.

In summary, axSpA has a significant burden and impact on an individual with this condition. It leads to significant functional disability, work instability, and other psychosocial impacts, resulting in reduced quality of life. The health economic impact, particularly on work participation and productivity, is considerable and provides a sound justification to improve modifiable disease parameters using effective therapies and a broad multi-disciplinary approach, which also needs to include employers and carers, in order to reduce this burden.

Key References and further reading

Barkham N, Kong O, Tennant A, ***et al.*** The unmet need for anti-tumour necrosis factor (anti-TNF) therapy in ankylosing spondylitis. *Rheumatology.* 2005;**44**(10):1277–81. doi: 10.1093/rheumatology/keh713.

Bedaiwi M, Sari I, Thavaneswaran A, ***et al.*** Fatigue in ankylosing spondylitis and nonradiographic axial spondyloarthritis: Analysis from a longitudinal observation cohort. *J Rheumatol* 2015;**42**(12):2354–60. doi: 10.3899/jrheum.150463.

Boonen A. A review of work-participation, cost-of-illness and cost-effectiveness studies in ankylosing spondylitis. *Nat Clin Pract Rheumatol.* 2006;**2**(10):546–53. doi: 10.1038/ncprheum0297.

Boonen A, Boone C, Albert A, *et al.* Understanding limitations in at-work productivity in patients with active ankylosing spondylitis: the role of work-related contextual factors. *J Rheumatol.* 2015;**42**(1):93–100. doi: 10.3899/jrheum.131287.

Brophy S, Davies H, Dennis MS, *et al.* Fatigue in ankylosing spondylitis: treatment should focus on pain management. *Semin Arthritis Rheum* 2013;**42**(4):361–7. doi: 10.1016/j.semarthrit.2012.06.002.

Cooksey C, Husain MJ, Brophy S, *et al.* The cost of ankylosing spondylitis in the UK using linked routine and patient-reported survey Data. *PLoS ONE.* 2015;**10**(7):e0126105. doi:10.1371/journal.pone.0126105.

Gran JT, Skonsvoll JF. The outcome of ankylosing spondylitis: a study of 100 patients. *Br J Rheumatol.* 1997;**36**(7):766–71. PMID: 9255111

Hamilton-West KE, Quine L. Living with ankylosing spondylitis: the patient's perspective. *J Health Psychol.* 2009;**14**(6):820–30. doi: 10.1177/1359105309341394.

Martindale J, Shukla R, Goodacre J. The impact of ankylosing spondylitis/axial spondyloarthritis on work productivity. *Best Pract Res Clin Rheumatol* 2015;**29**(3):512–523. doi: 10.1016/j.berh.2015.04.002.

National Institute for Health and Care Excellence: TNF-alpha inhibitors for ankylosing spondylitis and non-radiographic axial spondyloarthritis. NICE technology appraisal guidance [TA383]. Available at: https://www.nice.org.uk/guidance/ta383

Palla I, Trieste L, Tani C, *et al.* A systematic literature review of the economic impact of ankylosing spondylitis. *Clin Exp Rheumatol.* 2012;**30**(4 Suppl 73):S136–41. PMID: 23072824

Rafia R, Ara R, Packham J, *et al.* Healthcare costs and productivity losses directly attributable to ankylosing spondylitis. *Clin Exp Rheumatol.* 2012;**30**(2):246–53. PMID: 22409861.

Chapter 11

Imaging in axial spondyloarthritis

Key points

- Imaging has always been a key component in the diagnosis of ankylosing spondylitis as part of the modified New York criteria.
- With the increased availability of MRI and the development of the Assessment of SpondyloArthritis international Society axial spondyloarthritis (axSpA) criteria, there has been a shift from x-ray imaging of structural damage to MRI imaging of inflammation. This information can help in both the diagnosis of axSpA and in guiding treatment decisions in patients with this diagnosis.
- Imaging results must be evaluated in the context of the clinical picture and should not be acted on in isolation.
- Advances in technology are also likely to lead to the development of even better imaging modalities for axSpA in future.

Imaging has always played a key role in the diagnosis of ankylosing spondylitis (AS) and axial spondyloarthritis (axSpA). Historically, a diagnosis of AS required the demonstration of specific structural changes in the sacroiliac (SI) joints on x-rays in order to fulfil the modified New York (mNY) criteria. The subsequent Assessment of SpondyloArthritis international Society (ASAS) classification criteria for axSpA include an imaging and clinical arm (covered in more detail in Chapter 12), with the imaging arm incorporating both magnetic resonance imaging (MRI) and plain x-rays. In clinical practice, a diagnosis of axSpA usually involves identifying suggestive clinical features and characteristic radiographic lesions in the spine and SI joints, in addition to excluding alternative causes for the findings. In addition to diagnosis, imaging plays a role in monitoring the disease (see Chapter 13) as well as providing prognostic information. Classic radiographic features in axSpA include features suggestive of inflammation, osteodestructive changes such as erosions, and osteoproliferative (new bone) changes such as syndesmophytes and ankylosis in the vertebral spine. While chronic structural changes are best seen on plain radiographs (or computed tomography (CT) scans), acute inflammatory lesions can generally only be visualized by MRI. Nonetheless, the consequences of inflammation, such as sclerosis, erosions, and joint-space narrowing, can be detected on radiography, particularly in patients with long-standing disease.

Plain radiographs in axSpA

SI joint x-rays

Sacroiliitis is the hallmark of axSpA. X-rays can only detect chronic bony changes (damage) as a consequence of inflammation, but cannot indicate whether or not active inflammation is present. While a number of specific sacroiliac views have been proposed, none of these have been shown to be clearly superior and these x-rays can be difficult to interpret for those unfamiliar with such views. Therefore, standard antero-posterior views of the pelvis are recommended for imaging the SI joints as this modality also allows assessment of the hip joints, which are frequently affected in AS (see Figure 7.1)

While sacroiliac involvement is a relatively specific finding in axSpA, there is often a delay before structural changes can be visualized on plain x-rays. In a study of patients with newly diagnosed axSpA, radiographic sacroiliitis diagnostic of AS was seen in 33% of patients with a disease duration less than a year, 47% with a disease duration of 1–6 years, and 68% with a disease duration of 6–9 years, confirming that SI joint x-rays are mainly helpful in long-standing disease (Poddubnyy, 2012). It should be noted that the complex S-shaped anatomy of the SI joints, in which the direction of the joint space is oblique relative to the sagittal plane, and the inherent structural irregularities of the joint surfaces make the interpretation of radiographs difficult, and often leads to false-positive and false-negative readings, even among trained readers. The latest EULAR recommendations for the use of imaging in the diagnosis of axSpA still recommend conventional SI joint radiography as the first imaging method in patients with suspected sacroiliitis, apart from in young patients or those with short duration of symptoms, where MRI may be more appropriate (Mandl, 2015). However, some centres have moved to performing only MRIs in axSpA, but, as described elsewhere in this chapter, this only provides limited information on structural changes.

After obtaining a high quality film with good penetration, the individual SI joints should be inspected separately. Erosions appear as punched out lesions of the bone along the joint line, giving this an irregular appearance. The iliac side of the joint often shows changes first due to its thinner cartilage

Table 11.1 Grading of radiographic sacroiliitis

Grading of radiographic sacroiliitis	
Grade 0	Normal
Grade 1	Suspicious changes
Grade 2	Minimal abnormality – small localized areas with erosion or sclerosis, without alteration in the joint width
Grade 3	Unequivocal abnormality – moderate or advanced sacroiliitis with one or more of: erosions, evidence of sclerosis, widening, narrowing, or partial ankylosis
Grade 4	Severe abnormality – total ankylosis

compared to the sacral side. Accumulation of larger erosions can lead to the appearance of 'pseudo-widening' of the joint line. Reactive sclerosis often occurs adjacent to the joint line, both on the iliac and sacral sides. In later stages, partial and/or complete ankylosis ('fusion') occurs, and the joint line disappears. The radiographic changes of the SI joints are graded from 0 to 4, with each joint scored separately (grading criteria shown in Table 11.1).

While the mNY criteria required a patient to have either grade ≥2 bilaterally, or grade ≥3 unilaterally in order to fulfil a diagnosis of AS (see Box 12.1 and Chapter 12), in clinical practice, the presence of either sclerosis or obvious erosion, even in just one SI joint, is consistent with a diagnosis of axSpA in a patient with high pre-test likelihood of the disease and no suitable alternative explanation for these findings (for example, a 20-year old man with inflammatory back pain and uveitis).

Examples of SI joint x-rays with a range of grades are shown in Figures 11.1–11.4. However, it should be noted that scoring remains largely subjective, with significant inter- and intra-observer variability, even among experts. The practice of scoring SI joint x-rays in clinical practice has reduced significantly as this is no longer required for the use of biologics following the development of the ASAS criteria for axSpA.

Spine x-rays

While structural lesions in the spine are not part of the current axSpA classification criteria (see Chapter 12), characteristic spinal lesions can be seen on plain spinal radiographs. In about 5% of cases, these spinal changes can be seen even in the absence of radiographic sacroiliac changes. If performed, lateral radiographs of the cervical and lumbar spine are recommended. While thoracic spine involvement is common, thoracic spine x-rays are not

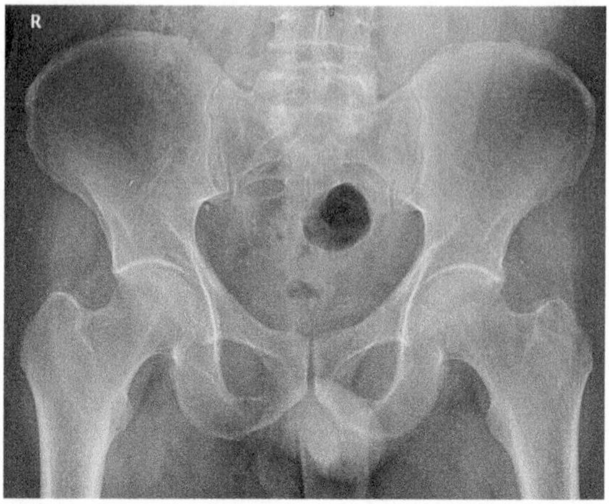

Fig. 11.1 Normal sacroiliac joint x-ray in a patient with axial spondyloarthritis. Grade 0 bilaterally.

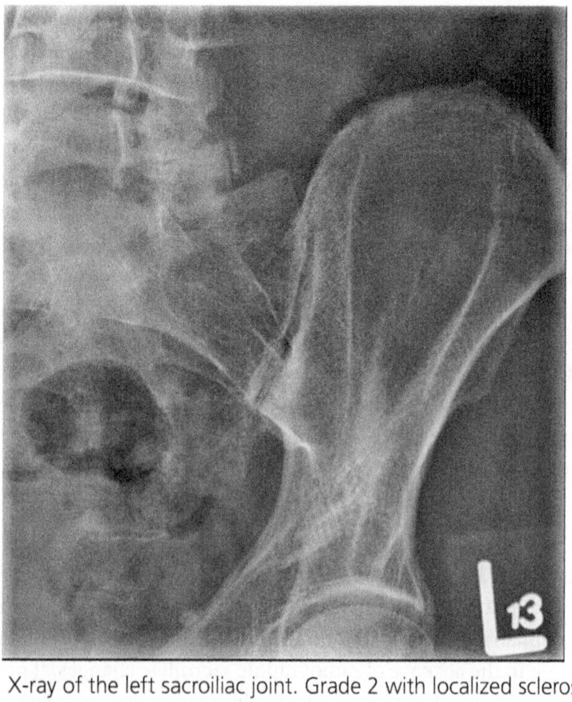

Fig. 11.2 X-ray of the left sacroiliac joint. Grade 2 with localized sclerosis and irregularity.

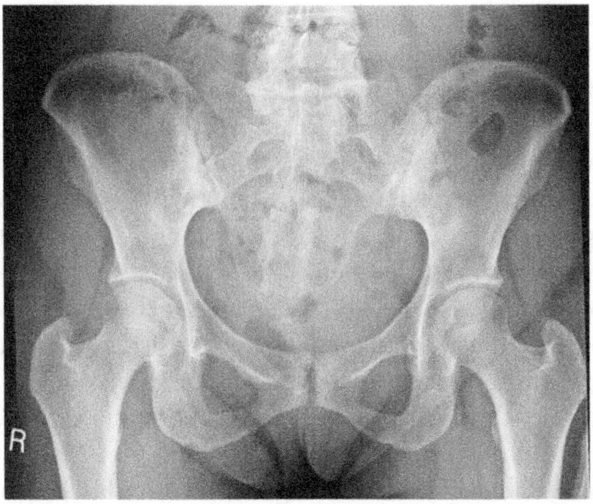

Fig. 11.3 X-ray sacroiliac joints with unequivocal sacroiliitis. Grade 3 bilaterally, with sclerosis, joint space narrowing and irregularity.

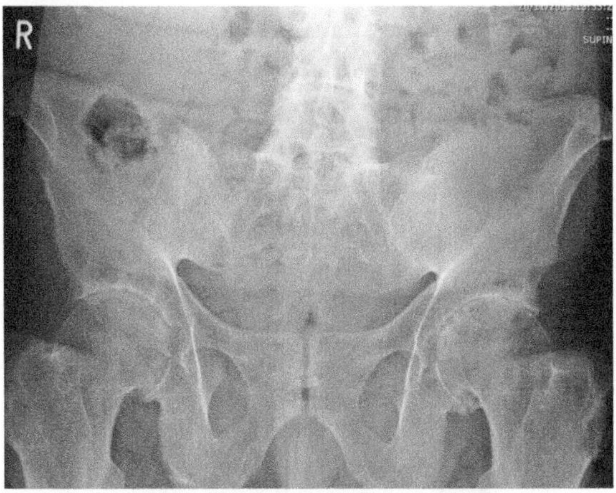

Fig. 11.4 X-ray sacroiliac joints with severe bilateral sacroiliitis. Grade 4 bilaterally with complete ankylosis. Note also concentric joint space loss in both hips.

routinely done due to the difficulty in detecting changes as a result of the overlying lungs and ribs. While the earliest spinal structural changes usually occur at thoraco-lumbar and lumbo-sacral regions, lesions can be seen at any level. There are certain pathognomonic changes on spinal x-rays that should be looked for in patients with axSpA.

The earliest x-ray changes occur at the antero-superior and antero-inferior margins of the vertebral bodies. At these sites, inflammatory enthesitis at the insertion of the outer fibres of the annulus fibrosus of the vertebral endplate leads to erosions of the vertebral corners, with secondary amorphous sclerosis, forming so-called 'shiny corners' or Romanus lesions. As more bone deposits around the end-plate, the normal concavity of the vertebral body is lost, leading to a squared appearance ('squaring' of the vertebrae).

The progression of the ossification of the outer fibres of the annulus fibrosus leads to characteristic thin, bony outgrowths between vertebrae termed syndesmophytes. These vertical outgrowths often begin at shiny corners. At least 50% of patients with AS develop syndesmophytes of the spine during the course of their disease. If disease onset occurs at a later age, the syndesmophytes may be laterally displaced due to a bulging annulus, and appear similar to, and difficult to distinguish from, the bridging osteophytes seen in degenerative disease. Examples of syndesmophytes in the lumbar and cervical spine are shown in Figures 11.5 and 11.6.

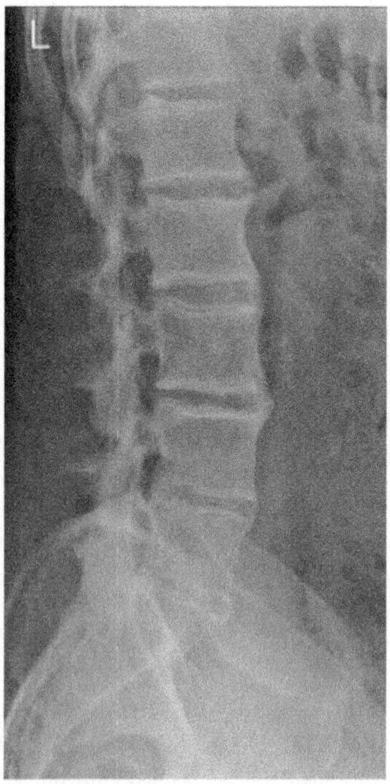

Fig. 11.5 Lateral lumbar spine radiograph showing widespread bridging syndesmophytes between vertebrae.

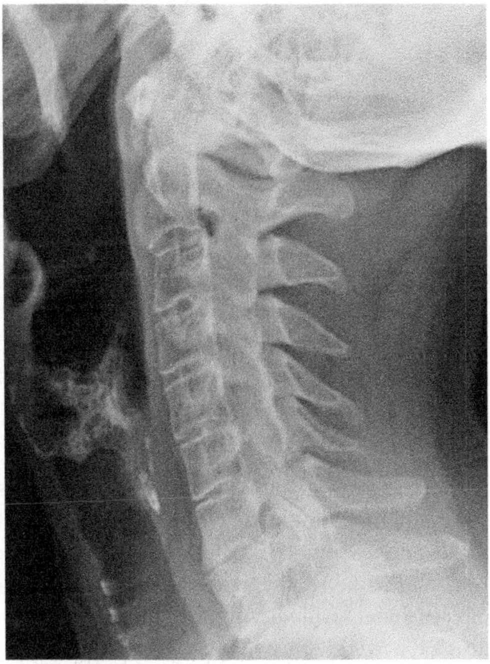

Fig. 11.6 X-ray of the cervical spine demonstrating fusion of the posterior elements in ankylosing spondylitis.

Other spinal elements such as the apophyseal joints, paraspinal ligaments, and spinous processes can also become ossified. Over time, in some patients, complete ossification and ankylosis can occur, leading to the signature radiographic abnormality of severe, late AS; the 'bamboo spine'. Fusion of the spinous processes can create a vertical stripe on frontal views of the lumbar spine, termed the 'dagger sign'. As the vertebrae and SI joints become ankylosed, the bony sclerosis seen in earlier stages disappears, likely due to immobility of the fused joints. An example of severe ankylosis of the spine, with superimposed pseudoarthrosis, is shown in Figures 9.2 and 9.3.

The progression to ankylosis of the spine generally occurs linearly over time; however, there is great heterogeneity and variability between patients (see Figure 11.7 for an example of radiographic progression over time). One study, which followed AS patients over a mean of 12 years, reported that a quarter of patients did not show any radiographic progression, a quarter developed clinically important progression (as quickly

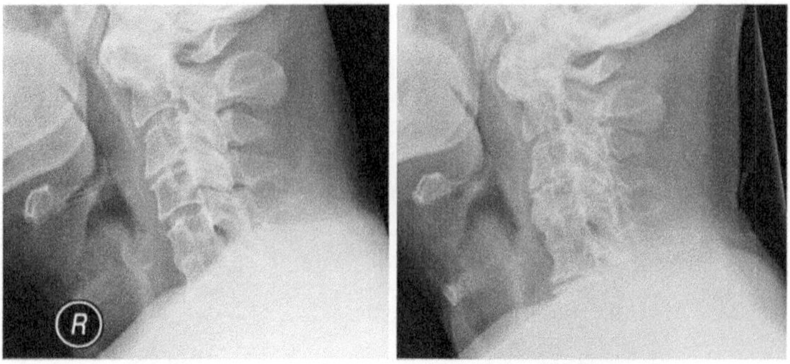

Fig. 11.7 X-ray of the cervical spine demonstrating progression in syndesmophyte formation and fusion over 5 years in a patient with ankylosing spondylitis.

as 2 years), and half showed a small amount of progression such as syndesmophyte formation, erosions, and squaring (Ramiro, 2015). Those with more progression were typically male, HLA-B27 positive, had a history of smoking, and had an increased amount of structural changes at baseline. Complete spinal fusion occurs in approximately 30% of patients who have had AS for over 30 years, and 40% of those with AS for over 40 years (Jang, 2011).

Scoring systems to quantify radiographic structural changes in the spine have been validated, but are mainly used for research purposes. The most commonly used is the Modified Stoke Ankylosing Spondylitis Spine Score (mSASSS), in which lateral views of the cervical and lumbar spine are graded, vertebra by vertebra, and scored based on the presence or absence of erosions, syndesmophyte formation, and ankylosis (Wanders, 2004). As disease progression is generally slow, radiographs of the vertebrae are usually not done more than every 2 years, unless there is clinical suspicion of another pathological process (such as fracture or 'pseudofracture' following trauma). The value of sequential spinal x-rays in clinical practice outside of clinical trials remains unclear and the practice is likely to reduce significantly with the availability of spinal MRI scans which avoid the radiation exposure associated with spinal x-rays.

In addition to the classic vertebral changes, up to 8–10% of patients with AS develop inflammation of the intervertebral discs, known as aseptic spondylodiscitis, or Andersson lesion. On conventional radiography, Andersson lesions are characterized by endplate erosions, sclerosis of adjacent bone, and disc calcification, with a normal or only mildly narrowed disc space. This lesion typically occurs in AS of longer duration, and can mimic infection (septic discitis), which usually requires MRI for differentiation (see Figure 11.12). Spinal fractures in AS may occur at the level of the disc or vertebral body and are covered in more detail in Chapter 9.

MRI in axSpA

Although conventional radiographic changes are used in the diagnosis of AS, MRI enables the detection of early disease, prior to the development of structural damage. MRI scans are particularly useful in detecting active inflammatory lesions, which has facilitated early diagnosis and greatly enhanced understanding of the course of axSpA. Generally, fat-saturated T2-weighted or, more commonly, short tau inversion recovery (STIR) MRI sequences are used to visualize active inflammatory changes. Inflammation appears as a high signal on these sequences, which are generally sufficient for this purpose. Therefore, the regular use of gadolinium or contrast is no longer recommended for routine diagnostic scans in axSpA. The characteristic axial inflammatory change seen on MRI in axSpA is 'bone marrow oedema' (BME) or 'osteitis' in the spine and SI joints. Histological correlation with bone biopsy of active lesions has confirmed inflammatory cell infiltrates (Bollow, 2000). Other inflammatory lesions frequently detected in axSpA on these sequences include capsulitis, synovitis, and enthesitis.

Chronic structural changes, such a fatty degeneration, are generally best visualized using T1-weighted sequences, although the diagnostic significance of these is currently unclear. While MRI scans can detect erosions and structural damage, x-rays and CT scans are generally superior for these chronic bony features of the disease. The typical MRI changes of the SI joints in axial spondyloarthritis are listed in Table 11.2.

Table 11.2 MRI lesions of the sacroiliac joints in axial spondyloarthritis

Typical MRI lesions of the sacroiliac joints	
Acute/ active inflammatory lesions	**Chronic inflammatory lesion**
◆ Bone marrow oedema/ osteitis	◆ Fatty changes/ fat metaplasia
◆ synovitis	◆ sclerosis
◆ capsulitis	◆ erosions
◆ enthesitis	◆ ankylosis
Best seen on STIR sequences	*Best seen on T1 sequences*

Most specialist units have developed standard protocols for MRI scans in axSpA, with scanning of the SI joints and whole spine recommended. These axSpA scans typically use T1-weighted (for chronic changes) and STIR or fat-saturated T2-weighted (for acute changes) sequences. In order to minimize scanning time, most protocols use 4 mm thickness semi-coronal sections of the SI joints, which usually generate 10–12 slices. Spinal protocols for axSpA generally involve sagittal slices of the thoraco-lumbar and thoraco-cervical spine. Although they can provide useful information, particularly about the posterior parts of the spine, axial or transverse slices are time-consuming and therefore not routinely done as part of diagnostic axSpA scans. There are a number of MRI scoring methods, but none of these are clearly superior or currently used in routine clinical practice. Extensive MRI inflammatory BME changes are associated with more inflammation and better clinical response to treatment with TNF inhibitors, so may be a useful prognostic indicator when making treatment decisions in axSpA.

MRI of SI joints

Active sacroiliitis in axSpA is characterized by subchondral and peri-articular high intensity BME adjacent to the SI joints on STIR and T2 MRI sequences (see Figure 11.8). In symptomatic patients, this subchondral BME generally correlates with elevated inflammatory markers. Specific definitions for active sacroiliitis have been formulated for use in classification criteria and are used in research settings. The definition of a 'positive MRI' is likely to evolve as MRI technology advances and further knowledge is gained about particularly the natural history of MRI changes in axSpA. The current ASAS expert consensus defines a positive MRI of the SI joints as one area of BME on two or more consecutive slices or two or more areas of BME on a single slice. An example of a positive MRI is shown in Figure 11.8. This definition of a positive MRI has recently been questioned by several investigators and is likely to alter over the next few years.

Other inflammatory findings that can be seen on MRI scans include synovitis, enthesitis, or capsulitis, although these have been less well studied than BME and are not diagnostic on their own. In addition, chronic structural lesions may be seen, such as sclerosis, erosions, fat deposition, and ankylosis. These chronic changes are generally best seen on T1-sequences, although MRI is not the optimal imaging method to assess structural changes, apart from fat metaplasia which is seen frequently (see Figure 11.9). As with all imaging, the results of MRI scans of SI joints should be assessed in the context of the clinical picture. Potential differential causes

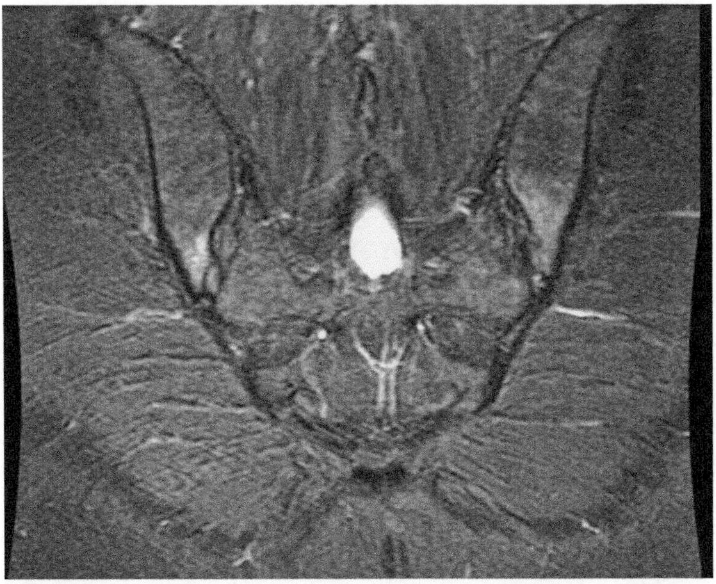

Fig. 11.8 MRI scan (fat-suppression) of sacroiliac joints with areas of bone marrow oedema (BME) in both sacroiliac joints (high signal). This single MRI image would meet the ASAS criteria for a positive MRI as there are two areas of BME on a single slice.

for apparent inflammation of SI joints on MRI include infection (which generally crosses anatomical borders unlike axSpA), sacral insufficiency fractures and osteosarcomas.

MRI of the spine

Active inflammatory lesions consistent with spondylitis can be visualized in the spine on MRI in those with normal radiographs, and infrequently in those with normal SI joint MRI imaging. Three phases of lesions have been described: active inflammatory lesions, post-inflammatory fatty bone degenerative lesions, and chronic structural change such as ankylosis. The characteristic acute inflammatory lesion is the Romanus lesion, also known the 'corner sign' or 'corner inflammatory lesion', which is a triangle-shaped BME lesion at one or more of the four corners of the vertebra. It is seen as high signal on sagittal views of STIR or T2-weighted images and is thought to correspond to enthesitis and osteitis at the attachment of the annulus fibrosus. Examples of characteristic corner

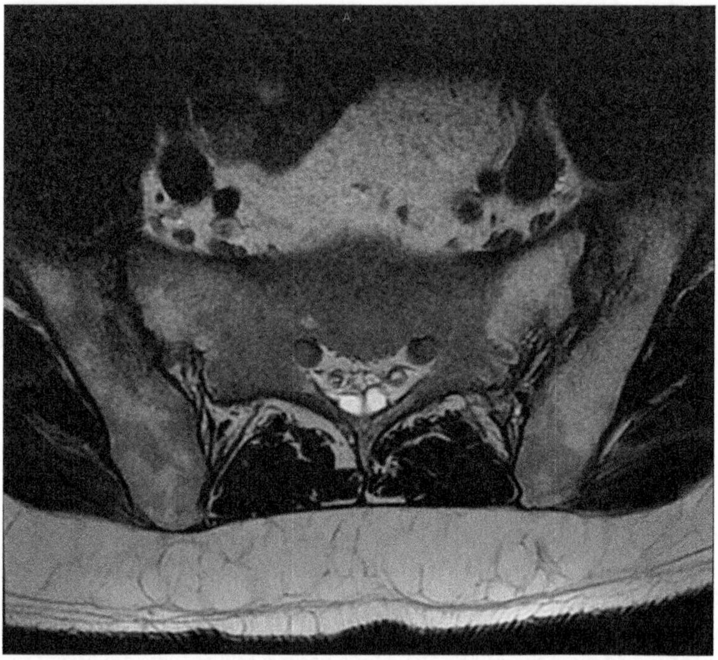

Fig. 11.9 Bilateral chronic changes of the sacroiliac joints on MRI scan (T1 sequence). There are extensive areas of bilateral fat metaplasia (fatty changes), as well as erosions and subchondral sclerosis.

inflammatory lesions on MRI of the lumbar and thoracic spine are shown in Figures 11.10 and 11.11.

Isolated corner oedema may however be non-specific, and most experts, including ASAS, consider active spondylitis in the spine to be present when there are three or more inflammatory corner lesions on at least two consecutive slices (sensitivity 81%, specificity 97% in those younger than age 40), although other definitions have also been proposed. Inflammatory BME changes may also extend into the pedicles and posterior elements of the vertebral column, which several studies have suggested may be highly suggestive of axSpA. Inflammation can also involve the intervertebral discs in aseptic spondylodiscitis (also called an Andersson lesion). This can lead to significant hyperintense signal on fat-suppressed MRI scans (see Figure 11.12) and needs to be differentiated from infective discitis, although this is usually possible on clinical assessment and imaging, without the need for tissue aspiration or biopsy.

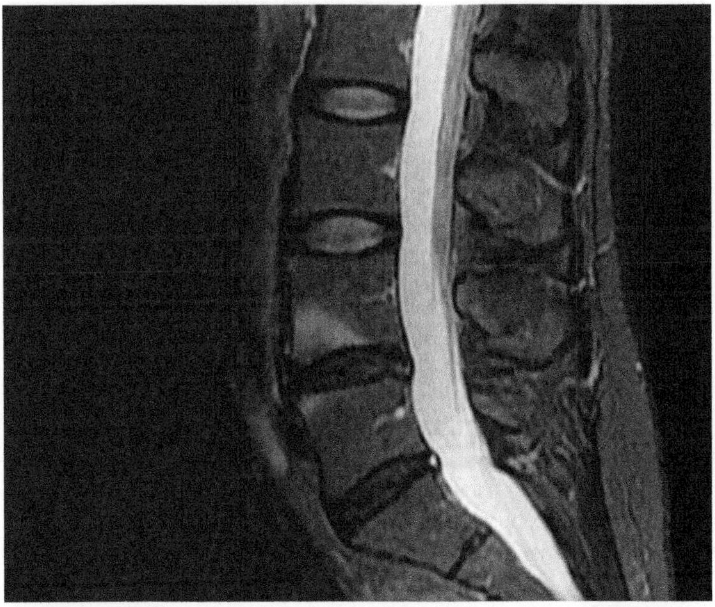

Fig. 11.10 Anterior corner inflammatory lesions (hyperintense) on STIR MRI scan of lumbar spine.

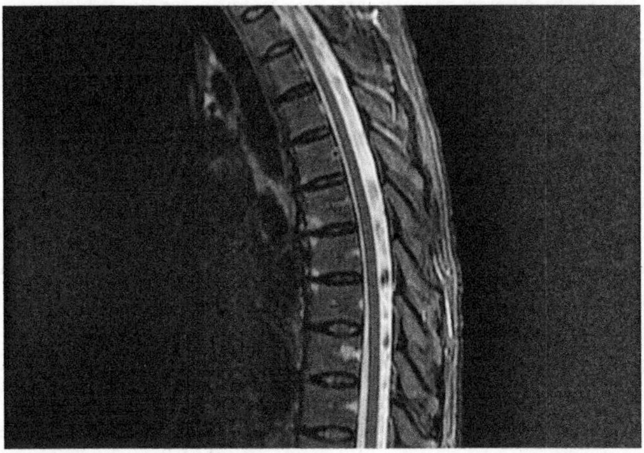

Fig. 11.11 Multiple anterior corner inflammatory lesions (hyperintense signal) in the thoracic vertebra on STIR MRI scan.

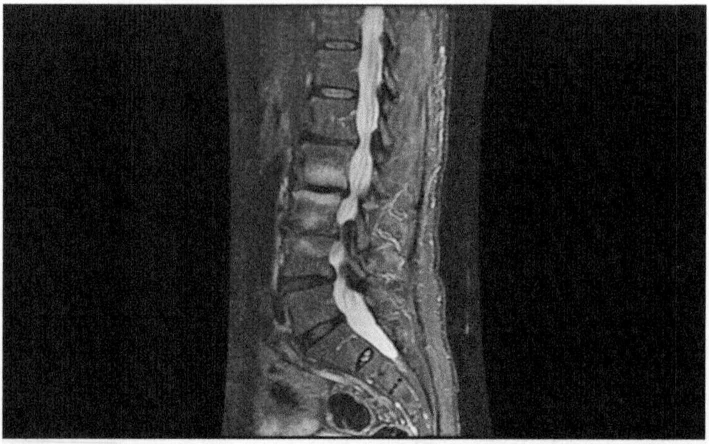

Fig. 11.12 MRI scan of lumbar spine in a patient with axial spondyloarthritis indicating hyperintense signal at L2/L3 on STIR sequence, consistent with inflammatory spondylodiscitis (Andersson lesion). While there are also some degenerative changes, note the relatively preserved disc height at this level.

Following the acute inflammatory phase, the Romanus lesion appears to be replaced by fatty tissue (fat metaplasia), which is apparent on T1 MRI sequences and can also manifest as a 'shiny corner' on plain radiographs. Fatty corner changes are less specific for axSpA than corner inflammatory lesions and are frequently also seen associated with degenerative disc disease. The formation of syndesmophytes has been reported to occur at inactive areas of apparent fat metaplasia. However, early syndesmophytes are not well visualized on MRI, and better assessed with radiographs or CT.

The diagnostic utility of spinal MRI in axSpA is still an evolving area and the current EULAR recommendations for imaging do not recommend the routine use of spinal MRI for the diagnosis of axSpA. However, this clearly depends on the clinical context and may be appropriate in cases where there is a high suspicion of axSpA, but no diagnostic SI joint MRI findings, and suggestive spinal MRI features that cannot be easily explained by other causes.

Other areas of axSpA involvement that may be seen on spinal MRI scans include the facet, sternocostal and costovertebral joints, again consisting of subchondral BME around the joints and synovial enhancement. Enthesitis of the anterior and posterior longitudinal ligaments is very common in axSpA and often associated with ligament thickening and adjacent BME.

The detection of active BME on MRI provides both diagnostic and prognostic value. Patients who have a high degree of spinal inflammation on MRI typically respond better to TNF inhibitor therapy than those with a lower degree of inflammation. In addition, the presence of both acute inflammatory and chronic structural changes on MRI at baseline appears predictive of the development of future structural changes.

Other imaging modalities in axSpA

CT scanning

CT scanning inherently has higher spatial resolution, making subtle erosions and subchondral sclerosis, particularly in the anatomically complex SI joints, easier to visualize (see Figures 11.13 and 11.14 for subtle and marked SI joint structural changes on CT scan, respectively).

Similarly, vertebral syndesmophytes are also better visualized with CT (see Figure 11.15 and 11.16).

The increased sensitivity and high degree of specificity compared to radiography makes CT the gold standard for detecting chronic structural change. However, CT is not typically used in clinical settings for this purpose as it involves a high degree of ionizing radiation, which is a particular concern in axSpA patients who tend to be younger. In addition, CT scans cannot detect active inflammatory lesions in the bone marrow or entheseal

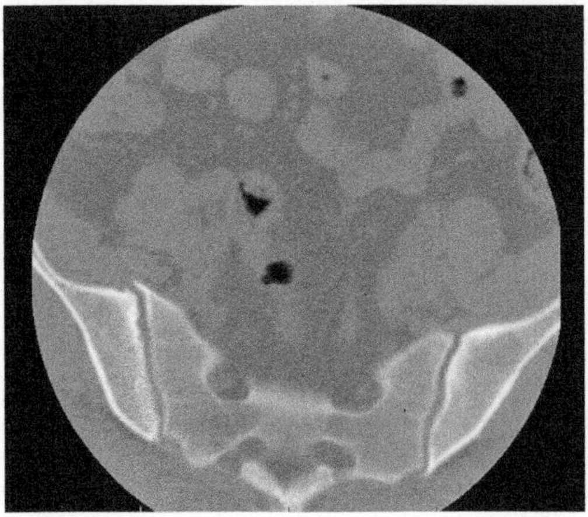

Fig. 11.13 CT scan showing subtle erosive change in the right sacroiliac joint, with mild sclerosis.

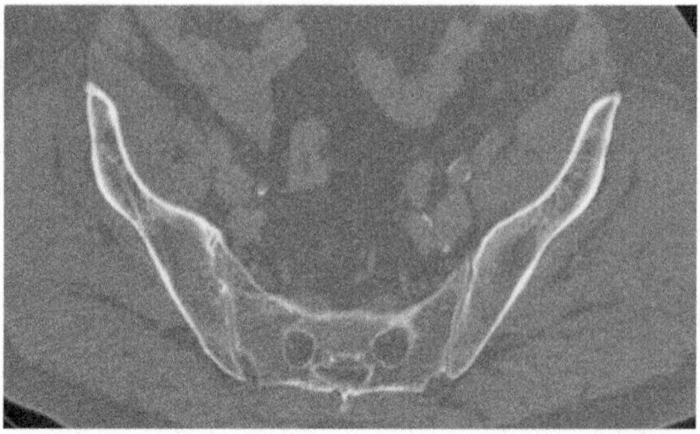

Fig. 11.14 CT scan evidence of joint space narrowing, anterior capsule calcification, and partial fusion of the right sacroiliac joint in a patient with ankylosing spondylitis.

sites, and are, therefore, not useful in early axSpA or in detecting active disease. Therefore, CT scans are only exceptionally used in axSpA to answer specific questions relating to structural changes (for example in planning for spinal surgery or where there is uncertainty relating to potential stress or spinal fractures).

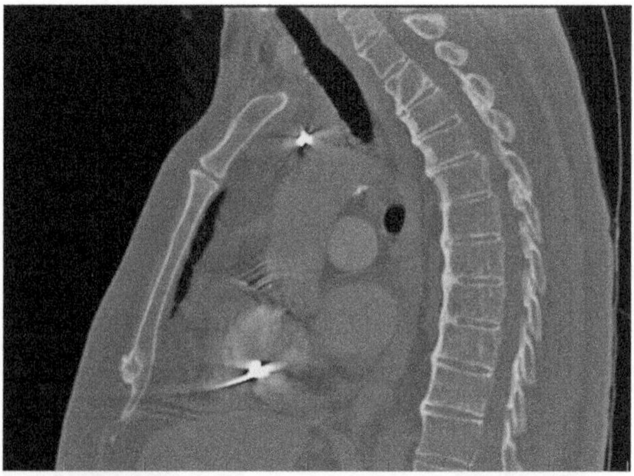

Fig. 11.15 CT scan evidence of anterior syndesmophyte formation and fusion of several thoracic vertebrae.

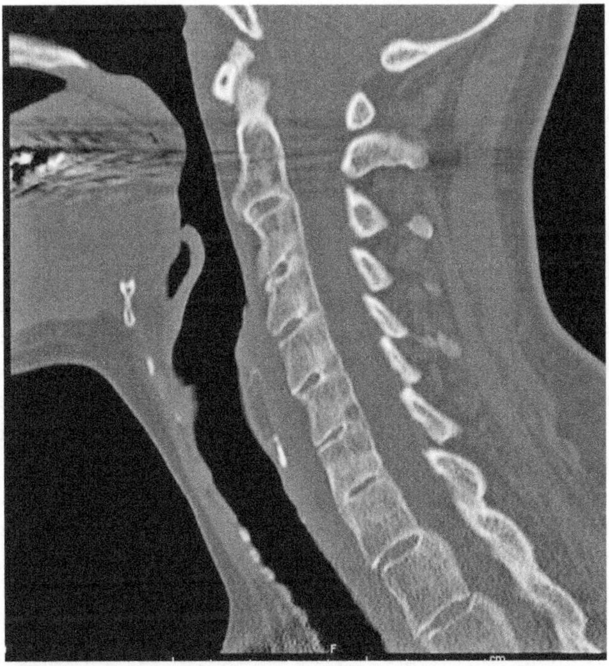

Fig. 11.16 CT scan of cervical spine demonstrating extensive posterior syndesmophytes and evidence of bony fusion in ankylosing spondylitis.

Bone scintigraphy (nuclear bone scans)

Scintigraphy was a technique traditionally used to evaluate spinal inflammation, particularly in early disease. While it is sensitive, with increased uptake in areas of inflammation, it is very non-specific and often over-reports minor degenerative changes as active sacroiliitis. With superior and safer techniques such as MRI now readily available, bone scintigraphy is not typically used in clinical practice anymore.

Imaging of peripheral musculoskeletal structures

Erosions may be seen on plain radiographs of peripheral joints in AS, but are far less common or severe than in patients with rheumatoid arthritis. Patients with axSpA can often have chronic swelling of the ankles, knees, and shoulder joints as part of their disease but only develop mild joint space narrowing after years of disease. In contrast, plain radiographs of the hip joints can show extensive osteodestructive changes, particularly in those with long-standing and more severe spinal disease, so these should always be actively inspected when reviewing pelvic films of SI joints (see Figure 7.1). The severity of hip arthritis may be measured using the Bath Ankylosing Spondylitis Radiology Index—hip (BASRI-h), in which the hips are each graded 0–4, with 0 being normal; 1, suspicious focal joint space narrowing (JSN); 2, mild circumferential JSN; 3, moderate JSN >2 mm or bone-to-bone apposition <2 cm; 4, severe bone deformity or bone-on-bone apposition of ≥ 2cm (Mackay, 2000).

In addition, osteoproliferative changes, including new bony formation and entheseal calcification, can occasionally be seen at peripheral sites. Entheseal structures, along the iliac crest and ischial tuberosity, can be become calcified into small enthesiophytes. While calcaneal spurs are commonly seen in spondyloarthritis (SpA), these are not specific and are also frequently seen as incidental findings on x-rays in those without disease (see Figure 7.4). Periostitis may also give a 'fluffy' or 'whiskered' appearance to bony margins at a number of sites, including the symphysis pubis, femoral trochanters, and other entheseal attachment sites, particularly of the lower extremities (see Figure 11.17). These findings are not specific for SpA and need to be interpreted in the context of the clinical picture. Dactylitis in SpA does not show bony changes on plain radiographs and generally requires high resolution MRI scanning to visualize.

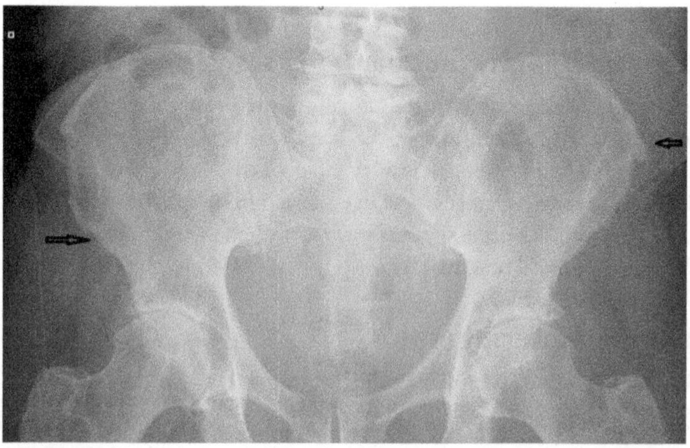

Fig. 11.17 Pelvic x-ray demonstrating 'whiskering' (depicted by arrows) of the pelvic brim due to enthesitis. Note also evidence of sacroiliitis and hip disease.

Ultrasonography of entheseal sites, particularly the Achilles enthesis, may reveal a thickened and hypoechogeneic tendon at its insertion into the calcaneus, with calcification, enthesophytes, and increased power Doppler signal. Ultrasound and MRI may also detect enthesitis or sub-clinical joint inflammation at a number of sites, thereby providing clinically useful information about disease activity. Studies have also looked into the use of ultrasound to detect active sacroiliitis, with mixed results. These ultrasound techniques require further validation before more widespread use can be recommended.

Future novel imaging modalities for axSpA

With technological advances, there are new imaging modalities emerging which may prove useful in the diagnosis and monitoring of axSpA in future. A number of these have shown promise in research settings, although their utility in daily clinical practice remains to be determined. Whole-body MRI allows the simultaneous assessment of inflammatory changes in the spine and peripheral sites, giving a better indication of overall disease activity. This technique may be particularly useful in future for screening at-risk individuals or for the initial evaluation of patients with axSpA. Diffusion-weighted and high resolution MRI may offer higher sensitivity for detecting inflammation or erosions than current conventional MRI. Advances in ultrasound technology, such as contrast-enhanced ultrasound and sonoelastography, may offer opportunities for improved assessment of peripheral enthesitis in axSpA. The increasing availability of positron emission tomography (PET) scans offers opportunities for very early detection of inflammation, particularly with the development of low radiation PET-CT and PET-MRI. The added value of PET over MRI alone remains to be determined to justify the added cost and radiation exposure, so this is likely to remain a research tool in most centres. Imaging developments are also advancing the evaluation of extra-articular manifestations and co-morbidities of axSpA, particularly for inflammatory bowel disease.

Summary

Imaging has always been a key component in the diagnosis and monitoring of AS. With the increased availability of MRI and the development of the ASAS axSpA criteria incorporating MRI findings, there has been a shift from x-ray imaging of structural damage to MRI imaging of inflammation. This information can help in both the diagnosis of axSpA and in guiding treatment decisions in patients with this diagnosis. However, imaging results must be evaluated in the context of the clinical picture and should not be acted on in isolation. There remains uncertainty about the natural history and the implications of certain MRI findings, which are likely to become clearer over the next few years, thereby facilitating incorporation of MRI changes into monitoring of disease activity in future. Advances in technology are also likely to lead to the development of even better imaging modalities for axSpA in future.

Key References and further reading

Bollow M, Fischer T, Reisshauer H, *et al.* Quantitative analyses of sacroiliac biopsies in spondyloarthropathies: T cells and macrophages predominate in early and active sacroiliitis- cellularity correlates with the degree of enhancement detected by magnetic resonance imaging. *Ann Rheum Dis.* 2000; **59**(2):135–40. doi: 10.1136/ard.59.2.135

Eshed I, Hemrann KG. Novel imaging modalities in spondyloarthritis. *Curr Opin Rheumatol.* 2015; **27**(4):333–42. doi: 10.1097/BOR.0000000000000186.

Hermann KG, Baraliakos X, van der Heijde DM *et al.* Assessment in SpondyloArthritis international Society (ASAS). Descriptions of spinal MRI lesions and definition of a positive MRI of the spine in axial spondyloarthritis: a consensual approach by the ASAS/OMERACT MRI study group. *Ann Rheum Dis.* 2012; **71**(8): 1278–88. doi: 10.1136/ard.2011.150680.

Jang JH, Ward MM, Rucker AN, *et al.* Ankylosing spondylitis: patterns of radiographic involvement–a re-examination of accepted principles in a cohort of 769 patients. *Radiology.* 2011;**258**(1):192–8. doi: 10.1148/radiol.10100426.

MacKay K, Brophy S, Mack C, *et al.* The development and validation of a radiographic grading system for the hip in ankylosing spondylitis: the bath ankylosing spondylitis radiology hip index. *J Rheumatol.* 2000; **27**(12):2866–72. PMID: 11128678.

Mandl P, Navarro-Compan V, Terslev L, *et al.* EULAR recommendations for the use of imaging in the diagnosis and management of spondyloarthritis in clinical practice. *Ann Rheum Dis* 2015;**74**(7):1327–39. doi: 10.1136/annrheumdis-2014-206971.

Poddubnyy D, Brandt H, Vahldiek J, *et al.* The frequency of non-radiographic axial spondyloarthritis in relation to symptom duration in patients referred because of chronic back pain: results from the Berlin early spondyloarthritis clinic. *Ann Rheum Dis.* 2012; **71**(12): 1998–2001. doi: 10.1136/annrheumdis-2012-201945.

Ramiro S, Stolwijk C, van Tubergen A, *et al.* Evolution of radiographic damage in ankylosing spondylitis: a 12 year prospective follow-up of the OASIS study. *Ann Rheum Dis.* 2015;**74**(1):52–9. doi: 10.1136/annrheumdis-2013-204055.

Wanders A, Landewé R, Spoorenberg A, *et al.* Scoring of radiographic progression in randomised clinical trials in ankylosing spondylitis: a preference for paired reading order. *Ann Rheum Dis.* 2004;**63** (12):1601–4. doi: 10.1136/ard.2004.022038.

Chapter 12

Classification criteria and diagnosis in spondyloarthritis

Key points

- The spondyloarthropathies (SpA) are heterogeneous multisystem disorders with no single 'gold standard' clinical, laboratory, pathological, or radiological feature to confirm the diagnosis. A number of criteria have therefore been developed to support clinical practice and research.
- The major SpA classification criteria include the modified New York criteria for ankylosing spondylitis (AS), the Amor and European Spondylarthropathy Study Group criteria for SpA and the Assessment in SpondyloArthritis international Society criteria for axial spondyloarthritis (axSpA). The evolution of these classification criteria has facilitated many significant advances in axSpA and SpA in general.
- The development of classification criteria for axSpA that do not rely on established radiographic damage has allowed biologic therapies to be investigated, and used, in earlier disease and for a wider population of patients.

The majority of chronic rheumatic conditions are heterogeneous multisystem disorders with no single 'gold standard' clinical, laboratory, pathological, or radiological feature to confirm the diagnosis. A number of criteria have therefore been developed to support clinical practice and research. Criteria have been particularly important for spondyloarthritis (SpA) as there is no associated serological test or obvious 'gold standard' definition. In this chapter, we review some of the major developments in classification criteria for ankylosing spondylitis (AS), axial spondyloarthritis (axSpA) and SpA.

Diagnostic versus classification criteria

Before considering the criteria developed for axSpA, it is important to note that there are significant differences between classification and diagnostic criteria. Confusion regarding the differences between these criteria has frequently resulted in the incorrect application of classification criteria in routine clinical settings, particularly relating to axSpA.

Diagnostic criteria are a set of symptoms, signs, and tests developed to guide the diagnosis of individual patients in routine clinical practice. In order to fulfil this purpose, diagnostic criteria must be broad and sensitive enough to encompass heterogeneity of the disease and identify as many patients as possible with the condition. Diagnostic criteria may allow flexibility in diagnosis, in that patients can be further divided as 'definite' cases when they fulfil all criteria, and 'probable' or 'possible' cases when they partially fulfil criteria.

In addition to 'pattern recognition', making a diagnosis in clinical practice often requires consideration of local factors (e.g. ethnic background, smoking rates) which influence the pre-test probability of a particular disease occurring in that geographical area. Furthermore, making a particular diagnosis requires other potential causes for the patient's symptoms, signs, or investigation results to be excluded, as far as possible.

The development and validation of diagnostic criteria is therefore challenging and requires different methods and reference standards to those used for classification criteria. There are only a few validated diagnostic criteria in rheumatology and the American College of Rheumatology has recently stated that it will no longer fund or endorse diagnostic criteria (Aggarwal, 2015).

In contrast, classification criteria are standardized definitions designed to create well-defined patient cohorts for clinical and epidemiological research studies. Classification criteria are intended to create relatively homogenous populations rather than capture the entire spectrum, or even majority, of patients who share a particular diagnosis or collection of features. Therefore, to avoid misclassification, these criteria require high specificity (low false positives) to prevent inclusion of patients without the disease, albeit at the expense of lower sensitivity (more false negatives). Not only do validated classification criteria allow comparison between different patient groups in a study, they also enable comparison of findings between different studies using the same classification criteria. However, the restrictive interpretation of disease may limit the external validity and ability to generalize to the wider population of patients in clinical practice who may have that particular diagnosis but not fulfil the more rigid classification criteria. Furthermore, classification criteria are context dependent (usually reflected in the stem component of the criteria) and cannot simply be applied to general populations.

It has been proposed that diagnostic and classification criteria may represent two ends of a continuum. However, the aims, development and utility of classification and diagnostic criteria differ significantly and, as such, these criteria cannot be applied interchangeably. Most importantly, diagnostic criteria essentially assume the diagnosis is unknown *a priori* and are designed to assist in establishing this in clinical practice, while classification criteria attempt to restrict the definition in a group of patients who are already assumed to have that particular diagnosis.

While classification criteria may provide some framework to aid in diagnosis and clinical decision-making in the absence of diagnostic criteria, they are inappropriate for routine use in daily clinical practice. As an example, if a patient has features that strongly suggest one particular diagnosis, and which cannot be explained by any other diagnosis, then the patient can usually be assumed to have that diagnosis, regardless of whether or not they fulfil the classification criteria. This patient would, however, not be eligible for participation in a clinical trial that is using those classification criteria as inclusion requirements. Similarly, there is a risk of misclassification, so classification criteria cannot simply be assumed to confirm a diagnosis in clinical practice. If a patient has features that fulfil specific classification criteria but which can also be explained by a number of other potential causes, then uncertainty about the diagnosis remains and further investigations may be required. For some conditions where aetiology is well defined (such as gout), diagnostic and classification criteria may be very similar and largely interchangeable. However, this is not the case for more complex and multifactorial conditions, such as axSpA. In axSpA, features vary between individuals, natural history is not predictable, features (and therefore certainty) vary with disease duration and investigations are also positive in a proportion of the normal population without the disease (e.g. HLA-B27, MRI changes).

In this context, it should be noted that the criteria for AS and axSpA are all classification criteria and not diagnostic criteria, so may guide but not define diagnosis in routine clinical practice.

Classification criteria for AS, SpA, and axSpA

In the early 1900s, AS was largely considered a 'subtype' of rheumatoid arthritis (RA) (see Chapter 2). However, it became increasingly apparent that AS was, in fact, more closely related to conditions like psoriatic and reactive arthritis than RA. The concept of seronegative SpA was established 40 years ago to characterize a distinct group of inflammatory arthritis with shared clinical features, radiological changes, HLA-B27 positivity, and familial clustering. At the time, five subsets were proposed: AS, psoriatic arthritis, reactive arthritis, enteropathic-related spondylitis and arthritis, and undifferentiated SpA. While this grouping was useful in clinical settings, the heterogeneity complicated the study of this disease group, particularly for the evaluation of the TNF inhibitors. Therefore, a number of classification criteria were developed in order to facilitate research into these diseases.

The most important classification criteria are covered here, with the main focus on the Assessment in SpondyloArthritis international Society (ASAS) criteria for axSpA. A number of criteria for the definition of inflammatory back pain (IBP) have also been developed and are covered separately in Chapter 6.

Modified New York criteria for AS

The most widely used classification criteria for AS are the modified New York (mNY) criteria (1984) (van der Linden, 1984). These criteria require at least one clinical criterion and a compulsory radiological criterion to be met in order for a patient to be classified as having 'definite AS' (Box 12.1). The clinical criteria relate to IBP, limited spinal mobility, and restricted chest expansion. The radiological criterion requires the presence of at least grade 2 sacroiliitis bilaterally or at least grade 3 sacroiliitis unilaterally on x-ray (see Table 11.1 for the sacroiliac grading scores).

Box 12.1 Modified New York criteria for ankylosing spondylitis (adapted from van der Linden, 1984)

Clinical criteria

- Low back pain and stiffness for >3 months, which improves with exercise but is not relieved with rest
- Limitation of motion of the lumbar spine in both the sagittal and frontal planes
- Limitation of chest expansion relative to normal values for age and sex

Radiological criterion (x-ray)

- Sacroiliitis grade ≥2 bilaterally or grade 3–4 unilaterally

Definite AS if the radiological criterion and ≥1 clinical criterion fulfilled.

Probable AS if only 3 clinical criteria present or radiological criteria present without any clinical criteria.

Source data from van der Linden S, Valkenburg HA, Cats A. Evaluation of diagnostic criteria for ankylosing spondylitis. A proposal for modification of the New York criteria. Arthritis Rheum. 1984; 27(4): 361–368

Although widely used in clinical and research settings for many decades, the mNY criteria have important limitations. Specifically, the focus is entirely on axial disease without taking any peripheral and extra-articular manifestations (EAMs) into account. Advanced radiographic sacroiliitis and clinical features, such as limited mobility and chest expansion, are typically late features of the disease that take several years to develop. Therefore, while these criteria are good for classifying established AS, they have low sensitivity in early disease and exclude patients who have not developed radiographic 'damage'. Furthermore, the scoring of sacroiliitis has been shown to have significant inter- and intra-observer variability, even among experts. Most importantly, there was an increasing recognition that many patients with classic clinical features never develop the advanced radiographic sacroiliitis required to fulfil these criteria.

Amor and ESSG criteria for SpA

In light of the heterogeneity of SpA, there was a desire to be able to define the wider SpA spectrum beyond the narrow radiographic definition of the mNY criteria for AS. In the early 1990s, the Amor criteria were developed to encompass all SpA subgroups without any pre-specified or compulsory entry requirements (Amor, 1990) (Table 12.1). Specifically, as radiographic features are not compulsory for the Amor criteria, patients with early SpA, previously termed 'undifferentiated SpA', could now be classified. These criteria consist of 12 items across four main domains: clinical, radiographic (sacroiliitis on x-ray), genetic (HLA-B27 or family history), and response to treatment (non-steroidal anti-inflammatory drugs). The clinical criteria include EAMs in order to capture the full SpA spectrum. Items are differentially weighted (range of 1–3); with radiographic sacroiliitis incurring the highest score (3) and a total score of at least 6 required to meet the criteria, with none of the items mandatory.

Shortly afterwards, the European Spondylarthropathy Study Group (ESSG) criteria were proposed (Box 12.2) (Dougados, 1991). The ESSG criteria required IBP and/or peripheral synovitis as entry criteria. Patients are classified as having SpA if they have at least one major entry criterion and one minor criterion from a list of seven items which include EAMs, family history, enthesitis, and sacroiliitis.

While the Amor and ESSG criteria had broader definitions of SpA, several clinical manifestations were not included, and the presence of sacroiliitis, a hallmark of axial disease, was not a mandatory requirement. These criteria, therefore, defined a more heterogeneous population of patients, which included purely peripheral psoriatic arthritis, reactive arthritis and enteropathic-related arthritis, in addition to those with axial disease. As such, their value in defining

Table 12.1 Amor classification criteria for spondyloarthritis (adapted from Amor, 1990)

Amor classification criteria for spondyloarthritis	Points
Clinical symptoms or past history of:	
Pain at night *or* morning stiffness of lumbar or dorsal spine	1
Asymmetrical oligoarthritis	2
Buttock pain	1
or if alternating buttock pain	2
Sausage-like toe or digit ('dactylitis')	2
Heel pain or other well-defined enthesiopathy ('enthesitis')	2
Iritis	1
Non-gonococcal urethritis or cervicitis, within 1 month before the onset of arthritis	1
Acute diarrhea, within 1 month before the onset of arthritis	1
Presence *or* history of psoriasis, balanitis, or inflammatory bowel disease	2
Radiological findings (x-ray):	
Sacroiliitis (bilateral grade ≥2 *or* unilateral grade ≥3)	3
Genetic background:	
HLA-B27 positive *and/or* family history of ankylosing spondylitis, reactive arthritis, uveitis, psoriasis, or inflammatory bowel disease	2
Response to treatment (non-steroidal anti-inflammatory drugs; NSAIDs):	
Clear-cut improvement within 48 hours after NSAIDs intake *or* rapid relapse of the pain within 48 hours after discontinuation of NSAIDs	2
A score of ≥6 is required to fulfil the Amor criteria for spondyloarthritis.	

Source data from Amor B, Dougados M, Mijiyawa M. [Criteria of the classification of spondylarthropathies] (In French). Rev Rhum Mal Osteoartic. 1990; 57(2): 85–9

disease populations for clinical trials was more limited, although they were helpful in estimating the true prevalence of SpA beyond just AS.

ASAS axSpA criteria

While the mNY criteria perform well in established disease, in most patients there is a delay of many years from the onset of symptoms until definite radiographic sacroiliac changes are detectable on plain x-rays. With the development

Box 12.2 European Spondyloarthropathy Study Group (ESSG) classification criteria for spondyloarthritis (adapted from Dougados, 1991)

Major criteria (require at least one of these)

- Inflammatory Spinal Pain or
- Synovitis – asymmetric or predominantly of the lower extremities

Minor criteria (require ≥1 of the following)

- Family history of ankylosing spondylitis, psoriasis, acute uveitis, reactive arthritis, inflammatory bowel disease
- Psoriasis
- Inflammatory bowel disease
- Preceding urethritis, cervicitis or episode of acute diarrhoea within 1 month before arthritis
- Alternating buttock pain
- Enthesopathy (lower extremity)
- Sacroiliitis on x-ray

A patient is classified as having spondyloarthritis if at least one major *and* one minor criterion is met.

Source data from Dougados M et al. The European Spondylarthropathy Study Group preliminary criteria for the classification of spondylarthropathy. Arthritis Rheum. 1991; 34(10): 1218–1227.

of potential disease-modifying therapies (biologics) for axial disease, there was a need to classify patients with axSpA earlier in the disease course. While the Amor and ESSG criteria allow earlier classification, the resultant SpA cohorts are too heterogeneous for use in randomized clinical trials testing a single intervention with a predefined primary endpoint in patients with predominantly axial disease. Furthermore, increased understanding and availability of magnetic resonance imaging (MRI) facilitated the detection of sacroiliitis and axial inflammation in patients without definite x-ray changes (see Chapter 11).

Experts from ASAS developed new classification criteria for axSpA which combined MRI evidence of inflammation with more traditional clinical, radiographic, and laboratory factors (Rudwaleit, 2009). The axSpA criteria require all patients to have chronic back pain of ≥3 month's duration with an onset before age 45 years. Patients with these entry criteria can then fulfil the ASAS axSpA criteria via one of two arms: the 'imaging arm' or the 'clinical arm' (Box 12.3 and Table 12.2).

Box 12.3 ASAS Classification Criteria for axSpA

In patients with chronic back pain (≥3 months) and age at onset <45 years

Imaging arm	or	**Clinical arm**
Sacroiliitis on imaging ◆ Positive sacroiliac MRI* *or* ◆ Definite radiographic (x-ray) sacroiliitis according to modified New York Criteria		HLA-B27 positive
Plus ≥1 SpA feature#		**Plus** ≥2 other SpA features#

#SpA features

Inflammatory back pain
Arthritis
Enthesitis (heel)
Uveitis
Dactylitis
Psoriasis
Crohn's/colitis
Good response to NSAIDs
Family history of SpA
HLA-B27
Elevated CRP

**Positive MRI: defined as active inflammation on MRI highly suggestive of sacroiliitis associated with axSpA*

Assessment of SpondyloArthritis international Society (ASAS) classification criteria for axial spondyloarthritis (axSpA). For a patient to be classified as having axSpA they must have chronic back pain (≥3 months duration) beginning prior to age 45 and fulfil either the imaging or clinical arm (adapted from Rudwaleit, 2009).

Table 12.2 Definitions of terminology used in ASAS classification criteria for axSpA (Rudwaleit, 2009)

Clinical criterion	Definition
Inflammatory back pain (IBP)	IBP according to ASAS experts criteria (see Box 6.4)
Arthritis	Past or present active synovitis diagnosed by a doctor
Family history	Presence in first-degree or second-degree relatives of any of the following: (a) ankylosing spondylitis, (b) psoriasis, (c) uveitis, (d) reactive arthritis, (e) inflammatory bowel disease
Psoriasis	Past or present psoriasis diagnosed by a doctor
Inflammatory bowel disease	Past or present Crohn's disease or ulcerative colitis diagnosed by a doctor
Dactylitis	Past or present dactylitis diagnosed by a doctor
Enthesitis	Heel enthesitis: past or present spontaneous pain or tenderness at examination at the site of the insertion of the Achilles tendon or plantar fascia at the calcaneus
Uveitis (anterior)	Past or present uveitis (anterior), confirmed by an ophthalmologist
Good response to NSAIDs	At 24–48 h after a full dose of NSAID the back pain is not present anymore or much better
HLA-B27	Positive testing according to standard laboratory techniques
Elevated CRP	CRP above upper normal limit in the presence of back pain, after exclusion of other causes for elevated CRP
Sacroiliitis by x rays	Bilateral grade 2–4 or unilateral grade 3–4, according to the modified New York criteria
Sacroiliitis by MRI	Active inflammatory lesions of sacroiliac joints with definite bone marrow oedema/osteitis suggestive of sacroiliitis associated with spondyloarthritis

Source data from Rudwaleit M *et al*. The development of Assessment of SpondyloArthritis international Society classification criteria for axial spondyloarthritis (part II): validation and final selection. *Ann Rheum Dis*. 2009;68(6);777–83.

ASAS axSpA criteria—imaging arm

To fulfil the imaging arm, a patient should have evidence of sacroiliitis, either on MRI images or on conventional radiographs, plus at least one of the predefined SpA features (Table 12.2). Definitions of 'positive' sacroiliitis on MRI have been developed by expert consensus (see Chapter 11). It should be noted that the current axSpA criteria include only sacroiliac MRI and not spinal MRI, and in the SI joints, only include active inflammatory (bone marrow oedema) but not chronic changes. Therefore, in routine clinical practice it is conceivable that a young patient with IBP may have no active sacroiliac MRI changes but have highly suggestive spinal and/or chronic MRI changes that cannot be explained by any other cause. This patient, therefore, almost certainly has a diagnosis of axSpA, but would not fulfil the criteria for the imaging arm of the ASAS axSpA classification criteria (see earlier comments in this chapter about the difference between classification and diagnostic criteria). Similarly, it has been suggested that up to 12% of healthy individuals may have MRI findings that could be construed to suggest 'active sacroiliitis'. Therefore, a 'positive' MRI alone in a patient with low pre-test probability for axSpA (e.g. other more likely explanation or preceding event) is not sufficient for making a diagnosis of axSpA. This again highlights how classification criteria cannot be relied on routinely for diagnostic purposes in daily clinical practice.

ASAS axSpA criteria—clinical arm

To fulfil the clinical arm, the patients fulfilling the stem requirements should be HLA-B27 positive and have at least two other pre-defined SpA features (see Box 12.3 and Table 12.2). There is no requirement for any imaging evidence of disease for the clinical criteria for axSpA. It should also be noted that IBP is considered as one of the 'optional' SpA features in the clinical arm, rather than an absolute entry requirement for these criteria, although all patients would have to have chronic back pain via the stem entry requirements.

Therefore, these ASAS criteria are intended to encompass the full spectrum of axSpA, ranging from those with established radiographic sacroiliitis (who can also be classified as AS) to those who have not developed radiographic x-ray sacroiliitis (referred to as 'non-radiographic axSpA' (nr-axSpA)). The term 'non-radiographic' was chosen in preference to 'pre-radiographic' as the latter suggests that all patients will progress to 'radiographic' AS, which is not the case (see Chapter 3 regarding natural history and radiographic progression). The nomenclature is, however, somewhat confusing and has led to misunderstanding among some clinicians who may incorrectly believe that non-radiographic refers only to the 'clinical arm' of the ASAS criteria. The term 'radiographic' applies to x-rays but not MRI, so is not interchangeable with 'imaging'. Therefore, the imaging arm includes patients with established radiographic changes, who would meet the mNY criteria for AS, and those with 'positive MRI' sacroiliac inflammation without the required level of sacroiliac x-ray changes, who are somewhat confusingly termed 'non-radiographic axSpA'. The clinical arm incorporates patients who do not fulfil the imaging arm but do meet the required clinical criteria. Therefore, the nr-axSpA group includes all patients in the clinical arm and those in the imaging arm with MRI inflammation but no sacroiliac x-ray changes.

The ASAS classification criteria for axSpA have a reported sensitivity of 82.9% and specificity of 84.4% overall (Rudwaleit, 2009). As such, the criteria perform better than the ESSG or Amor criteria, which were developed in the pre-MRI era of SpA. Not surprisingly, the more objective features in the imaging arm are associated with higher specificity (97.3%) but lower sensitivity (66.2%). It has subsequently been reported that using just the nr-axSpA imaging arm (MRI positive but no definite x-ray changes), the sensitivity is 57%, with the same specificity (Akkoc, 2015). The ASAS axSpA criteria have been suggested to have reasonable diagnostic utility in clinical settings, although the previously highlighted issues with using classification criteria in this setting need to be carefully considered. It should also be noted that in the absence of an unequivocal gold standard for the diagnosis of SpA, the development of these criteria relied on local expert opinion as the gold standard, which may have introduced bias. The criteria are, therefore, likely to require updating in future.

It should also be noted that the higher sensitivity and lower specificity of the clinical arm imply this group is more heterogeneous. This subgroup has raised particular concerns for the regulators and some clinical experts (Deodhar, 2014), and it should be noted that the TNF inhibitor licences for nr-axSpA currently apply to those patients with positive MRI and/or raised CRP; namely, those patients most likely to have both the condition and active inflammation.

Juvenile-onset AS

The mNY and ASAS axSpA criteria do not specify a lower age limit, so these could theoretically be used in children when they apply. However, the term juvenile-onset AS is traditionally used when the onset of symptoms occurs before the age of 16. The nomenclature in juvenile arthritis continues to evolve, so many of these patients have been variously classified as juvenile idiopathic arthritis (JIA), oligoarticular JIA, or enthesitis-related arthritis. It should be noted that there are significant differences between juvenile-onset and adult-onset AS. In contrast to the dominant axial disease in adults with AS, presentation with peripheral joint involvement is common in the juvenile-onset group. In particular, hip arthritis and enthesitis are frequently seen in juvenile-onset disease. Therefore, the ASAS axSpA criteria may not be as reliable in juvenile-onset AS and distinguishing this from other forms of juvenile arthritis may be difficult.

Furthermore, not all patients with juvenile-onset AS develop AS in adulthood, while 10–20% of people diagnosed with AS during adulthood report that their original symptom onset was before the age of 16. It has been suggested that the term 'juvenile AS' could be used to describe children who meet the criteria for AS before the age of 16 years and the term 'juvenile-onset AS' used to describe those whose symptoms began before age 16 but who do not fulfil the AS criteria until they are adults (Colbert, 2010). The nomenclature of juvenile-onset JIA is likely to evolve in future in response to changes in nomenclature in adult axSpA, as well as advances in imaging and understanding of the disease pathophysiology and natural history.

ASAS peripheral SpA criteria

To encompass the full spectrum of SpA, ASAS also developed classification criteria for peripheral SpA for patients with predominantly peripheral manifestations (Rudwaleit, 2011). A patient with arthritis, enthesitis, or dactylitis can be classified as having peripheral SpA, if they also have one or more of the pre-defined SpA features (such as uveitis, psoriasis) or if they have two or more of arthritis, enthesitis, dactylitis, previous IBP, or SpA family history (Figure 12.1). Unlike the ASAS axSpA criteria, which are limited to

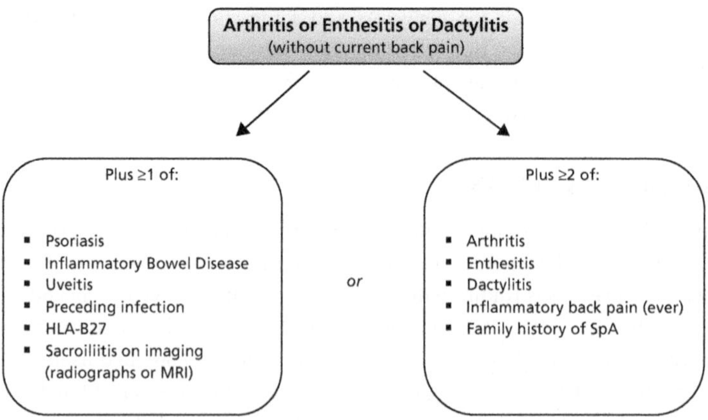

Fig. 12.1 Assessment of SpondyloArthritis international Society (ASAS) classification criteria for peripheral Spondyloarthritis (SpA) (adapted from Rudwaleit, 2011).

Source data from the Annals of Rheumatic Diseases, Rudwaleit M *et al.* The Assessment of SpondyloArthritis International Society classification criteria for peripheral spondyloarthritis and for spondyloarthritis in general. Vol 70, Issue 1, 2011

patients aged ≤45 years to reflect the younger age of onset of axial disease, the ASAS peripheral SpA criteria do not include any age restriction.

In patients with current IBP and concomitant peripheral manifestations, the ASAS axSpA criteria should be applied. While patients with psoriatic arthritis may be classified according to the ASAS peripheral SpA criteria, this is felt to be inferior to the more established CASPAR (for ClASsification criteria for Psoriatic ARthritis) criteria which remain the current standard inclusion criteria for clinical trials in psoriatic arthritis. Therefore, to date, the uptake and value of the ASAS criteria for peripheral SpA has been significantly more limited than the ASAS axSpA criteria.

Summary

In summary, the development and evolution of classification criteria has facilitated many significant advances in the field of axSpA and SpA in general. Specifically, the development of classification criteria for axSpA that do not rely on established radiographic damage (as required for the mNY criteria for AS) has allowed the efficacy of biologic therapies to be investigated, and confirmed, in earlier disease and for a wider population of patients.

However, there remains widespread confusion and misunderstanding about the role of classification criteria in the diagnosis of axSpA in clinical practice. The classification criteria for axSpA were not designed, and are inappropriate, for this purpose. In clinical practice, a diagnosis of axSpA should be made by physicians, ideally specialists with expertise in axSpA, considering all the features of an individual patient in the context of their local factors and potential alternative explanations in order to establish whether axSpA is the most likely diagnosis.

While it is possible to classify patients as having either AS or nr-axSpA, the consensus is that axSpA is a single disease entity containing some patients with clear structural damage (AS) and others judged to have no clear structural damage detectable on plain x-rays (nr-axSpA). It should also be noted that the cut-off between these two groups is completely arbitrary and patients in both groups may have a similar burden of disease (see Chapter 10). The natural history of the axSpA spectrum is still being determined, but it is increasingly clear that a significant proportion of patients with nr-axSpA will never go on to develop detectable structural damage (see Chapter 3). Furthermore, the patients with nr-axSpA who appear most likely to respond to treatment with biologic agents are those with positive MRI and/or elevated CRP. All these different criteria are based on dynamic concepts, and as our scientific understanding of SpA advances, definitions and criteria will need to be adjusted accordingly.

Key References and further reading

Aggarwal R, Ringold S, Khanna D *et al.* Distinctions between diagnostic and classification criteria? *Arthritis Care Res.* 2015; **67**(7): 891–97. doi: 10.1002/acr.22583.

Akkoc N, Khan MA. Looking into the new ASAS classification criteria for axial spondyloarthritis through the other side of the glass. *Curr Rheumatol Rep.* 2015; **17**(6): 515. doi: 10.1007/s11926-015-0515-2.

Amor B, Dougados M, Mijiyawa M. [Criteria of the classification of spondylarthropathies] (In French). *Rev Rhum Mal Osteoartic.* 1990;57(2): 85–9. PMID: 2181618.

Colbert RA. Classification of juvenile spondyloarthritis: Enthesitis-related arthritis and beyond. *Nat Rev Rheumatol.* 2010;**6**(8):477–85. doi: 10.1038/nrrheum.2010.103.

Deodhar A, Reveille JD, van der Bosch F *et al.* The concept of axial spondyloarthritis. Joint Statement of the Spondyloarthritis Research and Treatment Network and the Assessment of SpondyloArthritis international Society in response to the US Food and Drug Administration's comments and concerns. *Arthritis Rheumatol.* 2014;**66**(10):2649–56. doi: 10.1002/art.38776.

Dougados M, van der Linden S, Juhlin R *et al.* The European Spondylarthropathy Study Group preliminary criteria for the classification of spondylarthropathy. *Arthritis Rheum.* 1991;**34**(10):1218–27. doi: 10.1002/art.1780341003

Rudwaleit M, van der Heijde D, Landewé R *et al.* The development of Assessment of SpondyloArthritis international Society classification criteria for axial spondyloarthritis (part II): validation and final selection. *Ann Rheum Dis.* 2009;**68**(6);777–83. doi: 10.1136/ard.2009.108233.

Rudwaleit M, van der Heijde D, Landewé R, *et al.* The Assessment of SpondyloArthritis International Society classification criteria for peripheral spondyloarthritis and for spondyloarthritis in general. *Ann Rheum Dis.* 2011; **70**(1):25–31. doi: 10.1136/ard.2010.133645.

Sieper J, Rudwaleit M, Baraliakos X *et al.* The Assessment of SpondyloArthritis international Society (ASAS) handbook: a guide to assess spondyloarthritis. *Ann Rheum Dis.* 2009;**68**(Suppl II):ii1–44. doi:10.1136/ard.2008.104018.

van der Linden S, Valkenburg HA, Cats A. Evaluation of diagnostic criteria for ankylosing spondylitis. A proposal for modification of the New York criteria. *Arthritis Rheum.* 1984;**27**(4):361–8. doi: 10.1002/art.1780270401.

Zeidler H, Amor B. The Assessment in Spondyloarthritis International Society (ASAS) classification criteria for peripheral spondyloarthritis and for spondyloarthritis in general: the spondyloarthritis concept in progress. *Ann Rheum Dis.* 2011; **70**(1): 1–3. doi: 10.1136/ard.2010.135889.

Chapter 13

Assessment and monitoring outcomes in axial spondyloarthritis

Key points

- Axial spondyloarthritis (axSpA) is a heterogeneous condition with multiple effects and a variable course. Monitoring outcomes is required to optimize treatment and care.
- Monitoring outcomes in routine clinical practice has resource and logistic implications, so clinicians and teams looking after patients with axSpA need to determime which aspects they will monitor locally.
- Suggested key validated outcomes for axSpA include a range of patient-reported and clinician-assessed measures covering disease activity, symptoms (such as pain, stiffness, and fatigue), function, mobility, work disability, and quality of life.
- Most national and international guidelines for the use of biologics require regular monitoring of disease activity.

Axial spondyloarthritis (axSpA) is a chronic condition with a variable course and, as such, requires regular assessment to monitor disease activity, functional status, disease progression, and response to therapy in order to inform treatment decisions and optimize care. Monitoring outcomes ensures that patients who progress rapidly or who develop extra-articular manifestations (EAMs) can be identified early and treated appropriately.

ASAS core datasets and monitoring in clinical practice

The absence of reliable biomarkers of disease activity and prognosis has led to the development of a large number of validated outcome measures, many of which are patient reported. While the use of outcome measures is well established in clinical trials, the regular use of assessments in routine clinical practice was limited until the introduction of the TNF inhibitors, which necessitated regular monitoring to evaluate their efficacy and justify the use of these expensive drugs. In response to this requirement, the Assessment of SpondyloArthritis international Society (ASAS) defined specific core sets of measurement domains in order to standardize the monitoring patients with axSpA in daily clinical practice outside of clinical trials (Sieper, 2009). The core set was developed using consensus expert opinion based on literature review and clinical experience. The ASAS core set was grouped to cover three progressive clinical situations: (1) symptom modifying anti-rheumatic drugs (SM-ARDs) and physiotherapy, (2) clinical record keeping, and (3) disease-controlling anti-rheumatic treatment (DC-ART) (Table 13.1). The level and frequency of core monitoring would therefore be based on the patient's disease severity and current treatments, with those patients receiving DC-ARTs (effectively biologic therapies) undergoing the highest level of monitoring incorporating all three domains. In daily clinical practice, the

Table 13.1 ASAS/OMERACT core domains for ankylosing spondylitis (Sieper, 2009)

Domain	Instrument
Symptom-modifying anti-rheumatic drugs (SM-ARDs) or physiotherapy	
Physical function	BASFI
Spinal stiffness	NRS/VAS
Patient global assessment	NRS/VAS
Spinal mobility	BASMI *or* chest expansion, modified Schober, occiput to wall, cervical rotation, and lateral spinal flexion
Fatigue	Fatigue question on BASDAI
Pain	NRS/VAS for pain
Clinical record keeping (in addition to the above)	
Acute phase reactants	CRP or ESR
Peripheral joints/ entheses	Validated enthesitis score
Disease-controlling anti-rheumatic treatments (DC-ART) (in addition to the above)	
Spine radiographs	Lateral lumbar and cervical spine

Source data from Sieper J, Rudwaleit M, Baraliakos X et al. The Assessment of SpondyloArthritis international Society (ASAS) handbook: a guide to assess spondyloarthritis. Ann Rheum Dis. 2009; 68(Suppl II): ii1–ii44.

level of monitoring is driven largely by availability of resources to perform monitoring (e.g. physiotherapists/metrologists, specialist axSpA clinics) and the relevant funders' or regulators' requirements for the monitoring of biologic therapies in axSpA. Furthermore, while many of these outcomes are patient-reported or can be collected by allied healthcare professionals (e.g. physiotherapists or nurses), detailed clinical assessment by specialist physicians (e.g. rheumatologist) is still required, particularly in patients with complex disease and those on biologics. Furthermore, input from specialists in other disciplines (e.g. gastroenterology, ophthalmology) is also required for those patients with EAMs (covered in Chapter 8).

This chapter will focus largely on the assessment and monitoring of patients with axSpA in clinical practice, particularly the monitoring of patients receiving biologic therapies (the drug treatments are covered in Chapter 15). Regular longitudinal measurement and recording of outcomes facilitates not only the assessment of response to therapy, but also allows a long-term picture of the patient's disease, and impact thereof, to be developed. This is particularly important in slowly progressive and heterogeneous conditions like axSpA. Patient-reported outcome measures also enable the patient to participate more actively in the management of their own disease. It should be noted that most instruments were developed for ankylosing spondylitis (AS) prior to the development of the ASAS classification criteria for axSpA, but have largely been adapted for use across the axSpA spectrum in clinical practice and trials. Furthermore, many of the instruments were initially developed as visual analogue scales (VAS) but have subsequently been adapted as numerical rating scales (NRS) in order to facilitate their ease of use in busy clinical settings and avoid some of the technical issues related to inconsistencies in VAS line lengths when copied. Electronic versions of most patient-reported tools are also being increasingly developed and used in clinical practice.

Modern clinical assessment in axSpA includes a combination of patient self-reported instruments, clinician-measured outcomes, clinical examination, laboratory tests, and imaging. For ease of reference, the assessments are considered in this chapter according to the component of axSpA that is being measured, rather than according to methodology.

Disease activity

Bath Ankylosing Spondylitis Disease Activity Index

The Bath Ankylosing Spondylitis Disease Activity Index (BASDAI) is a self-administered composite index for the assessment of disease activity. It comprises six questions and covers three aspects which together reflect disease

Table 13.2 BASDAI questions and domains

Patients are asked to answer each of the following relating to the *past week*: (each question is answered on 100 mm visual analogue scale or numerical rating scale; range from 'none' to 'very severe', except question 6)

Specific question on BASDAI instrument	Domain being tested
How would you describe the overall level of fatigue/tiredness you have experienced?	Fatigue
How would you describe the overall level of AS neck, back or hip pain you have had?	Spinal pain
How would you describe the overall level of pain/swelling in joints other than neck, back, or hips you have had?	Peripheral arthritis
How would you describe the overall level of discomfort you have had from any areas tender to touch or pressure?	Enthesitis
How would you describe the overall level of morning stiffness you have had from the time you wake up?	Intensity of morning stiffness
How long does your morning stiffness last from the time you wake up? (range 0-2 hours or more)	Duration of morning stiffness

BASDAI calculation = ((Q5 + Q6)/2 + Q1 + Q2 + Q3 + Q4)/5

activity, namely stiffness, pain, and fatigue, over the past week (Table 13.2). The score is obtained using either a 100 mm VAS or 0–10 NRS for each of the six scales, with the final score then calculated by taking the average of questions 5 and 6 (relating to morning stiffness), adding this to the other four question scores and then dividing by 5. The result is a score ranging from 0 to 10, with higher scores representing higher disease activity. The BASDAI is a key measurement when making treatment decisions regarding TNF inhibitors, with a BASDAI score ≥4 generally indicating high disease activity and those in whom a TNF blocker might be appropriate. The smallest important measurable difference (minimal clinically important difference; MCID) in BASDAI is thought to be 1, on a scale of 0–10. Most rheumatology departments will monitor BASDAI at every clinical visit.In the absence of disease flares or changes in treatment, the BASDAI has demonstrated good stability over time, allowing it to be used to monitor longitudinal disease activity and treatment response. However, concerns have been raised regarding the validity of the BASDAI in the measurement of active inflammation in axSpA. BASDAI lacks an objective marker of disease activity, such as the C-reactive protein (CRP) in the 28 joint disease activity score (DAS28) used in rheumatoid arthritis (RA). Studies have shown poor correlation between BASDAI, inflammation on magnetic resonance imaging (MRI) scans, and acute phase reactants (such as CRP). Furthermore, the BASDAI score can also be high in patients with pain due to other causes, such as mechanical back pain or fibromyalgia, and is influenced by factors such as anxiety, depression, and general health status unrelated to axSpA.

Acute phase reactants

While the acute phase reactants CRP and erythrocyte sedimentation rate (ESR) are key measures of disease activity in other forms of inflammatory arthritis, particularly RA, they have been less useful in AS. A significant proportion of patients with only axial disease will never have a raised CRP. Furthermore, studies of non-steroidal anti-inflammatory drugs in AS did not demonstrated significant reduction in CRP despite improvement in patient-reported outcomes such as the BASDAI. CRP and ESR are more likely to be raised in patients with peripheral arthritis or significant underlying inflammatory bowel disease. The acute phase reactants had therefore largely fallen out of favour for monitoring disease activity of AS in clinical practice.

With the advent of the effective biologic therapies which demonstrate reduction in CRP, particularly high sensitivity CRP, and the recognition that CRP can be an objective measure of inflammation in some axSpA patients, there has been renewed interest in monitoring acute phase reactants in clinics. ESR has not been found to be superior to CRP in assessing disease activity, with no additive benefit of measuring both markers. The choice of acute phase reactant is, therefore, often based on local availability and protocols. Where this is not an issue, there has been a move towards CRP being the preferred marker as it has been identified as a predictor of response to biologic treatments in axSpA (see Chapter 15) and raised CRP at baseline is associated with a greater burden of radiographic damage in AS. As part of these developments, the acute phase reactants have also been incorporated into the newer composite disease activity scores.

Ankylosing Spondylitis Disease Activity Score

Concerns about the BASDAI led to the development of the Ankylosing Spondylitis Disease Activity Score (ASDAS). The ASDAS is a composite five-item instrument incorporating three components of the BASDAI (spinal

Table 13.3 Parameters for ASDAS

Parameters	**Source**
1. Total spinal pain	BASDAI question 2 (see Table 13.2)
2. Patient global disease activity	BAS-G/PGA (see Table 13.4)
3. Peripheral pain/swelling	BASDAI question 3 (see Table 13.2)
4. Duration of morning stiffness	BASDAI question 6 (see Table 13.2)
5. CRP (in mg/l) or ESR	Laboratory test

ASDAS calculator available on the ASAS website (www.asas-group.org)

pain, peripheral joint pain/swelling, and duration of morning stiffness), the patient global assessment of disease activity, and acute phase reactant result (CRP or ESR) (Table 13.3). A complex formula is used to give each individual component a relative weighting, depending on the importance of the item. A number of online ASDAS calculators are available, including on the ASAS website (www.asas-group.org). The instrument has been validated and performed well in a number of different studies.

Validated cut off values for disease activity states and improvement criteria have subsequently been defined for the ASDAS (Figure 13.1). These ASDAS

(A) Cut-offs for disease activity state using ASDAS

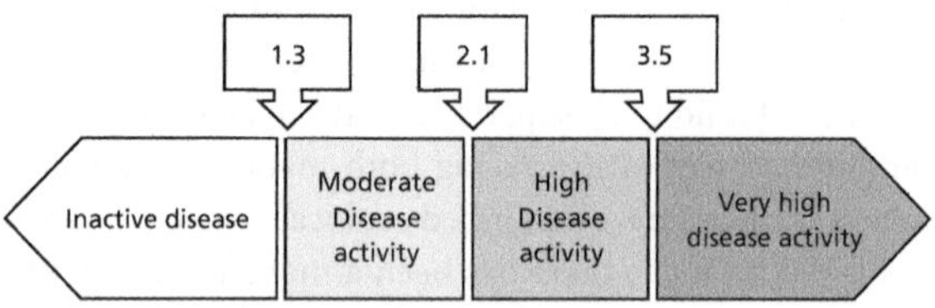

(B) Cut-offs for response definitions using ASDAS

Response or improvement	**ASDAS change**
Clinically important improvement	Change in ASDAS of ≥ 1.1 from baseline
Major improvement	Change in ASDAS of ≥ 1.1 from baseline

Fig. 13.1 Cut-off values for the ASDAS (adapted from Machado, 2011).

Source data from Machado P, Landewe R, Lie E, et al. Ankylosing Spondylitis Disease Activity Score (ASDAS): defining cut-off values for disease activity states and improvement scores. Ann Rheum Dis. 2011; 70(1): 47–53 cut-offs allow the patient to be categorized into one of four disease activity states: inactive disease, moderate disease activity, high disease activity, and very high disease activity (Machado, 2011). ASDAS improvement scores have also been defined for: clinically important improvement and major improvement.

While familiarity and ease-of-use mean BASDAI is still the dominant instrument currently used in clinical practice to measure disease activity, the higher discriminatory capacity of ASDAS and ability to better assess the disease activity state and clinically meaningful improvement will undoubtedly lead to increased use of this instrument in future. For these reasons, ASDAS is also likely to feature increasingly in clinical trials in axSpA, although use as primary outcome measure in phase III trials would also require acceptance and approval by the drug regulators.

ASAS response rates

ASAS has also defined criteria for defining response to treatment (e.g. ASAS20, ASAS40, partial remission), which are used as key outcome measures in clinical trials. The ASAS20 response rate has been the most commonly used primary outcome measure in the TNF inhibitor clinical trials (see Chapter 15 and Table 15.3). An ASAS20 response is defined as an improvement with treatment of ≥20% and an absolute improvement of at least one unit, compared to baseline, in at least three of the following four domains, with no worsening in the remaining domain: physical function (measured by BASFI), spinal pain, patient global disease assessment, and inflammation (derived from questions 5 and 6 of BASDAI). These ASAS response rates (number or proportion of patients achieving a pre-specified ASAS response) are intended for groups of patients, rather than individual patients, in order to allow comparison between different interventions in clinical trials. As such, these measures are not recommended or intended for use in monitoring of an individual with axSpA in daily clinical practice.

Spinal pain and stiffness

Pain and stiffness in the spine are the prototypic features experienced by patients with AS. The ASAS core domains specify monitoring both general and nocturnal spinal pain in patients with axSpA. This allows the diurnal variation associated with back pain in axSpA to be captured, but in practice many departments simply use a single measure of general spinal pain. This is self-administered using either a VAS or NRS to give a score for spinal pain, over the past week, ranging from 0 to 10, where 0 is 'no pain' and 10 is 'most severe pain'. Longitudinal spinal pain scores are useful to chart an individual patient's pain over time, although the MCID is unknown. The spinal pain score does not distinguish other causes of pain, which often limit its utility in monitoring response to therapy in clinical practice.

Spinal stiffness is generally assessed using the questions about morning stiffness in the BASDAI. Morning stiffness is felt to reflect inflammation and should be distinguished from reduced spinal mobility or range of movement due to structural damage such as syndesmophytes and ankylosis. The former generally is generally worse in the morning with diurnal variation, while the latter is largely unchanged throughout the day with no improvement with activity.

Global disease scores

Patient global scores are essentially objective measures of the standard greeting question 'How are you feeling?' which attempt to capture both the patient's overall perception of their disease status, as well as how this is affecting their life.

Patient Global Assessment

The Patient Global Assessment (PGA) is a simple self-administered measure and is generally considered as the single best measure for use in clinical practice. The PGA asks 'How active was your spondylitis on average over the last week?' which is captured on a single VAS or NRS.

Bath Ankylosing Spondylitis Global score

The Bath Ankylosing Spondylitis Global score (BAS-G) is an alternative instrument and essentially captures average well-being over both the past week and the past 6 months (see Table 13.4 for a comparison of the PGA and BAS-G).

Table 13.4 Comparison of PGA and BAS-G

	PGA	BAS-G
Specific question	How active was your spondylitis on average during the last week?	How have you been over the last week? How have you been over the past 6 months?
Response range	'not active' to 'very active'	'very good' to 'very bad'
Measurement	Single NRS/VAS	Average of two NRS/VAS

Both global measures have demonstrated good response to change. While more comprehensive quality of life measures are available for axSpA, the patient global assessments are felt to be good indicators of disease-related quality of life and more practical to administer in clinical practice. A patient global assessment is also required for the ASDAS composite score.

Physical function

Bath Ankylosing Spondylitis Functional Index

The Bath Ankylosing Spondylitis Functional Index (BASFI) is a patient-reported instrument consisting of 10 questions asking a patient to define the level of difficulty in performing certain specific and general day-to-day tasks (Box 13.1). The BASFI questions focus particularly on activities reflecting spinal function, as opposed to more generic functional questionnaires which may underestimate the functional impact of spinal involvement. Each activity is graded from easy to impossible using a 0–100 VAS or 0–10 NRS. The final BASFI score is the average of the individual scores, with higher scores representing more severe functional impairment.

Box 13.1 Activities measured by BASFI

The patient is asked to each of the following activities on a VAS/NRS ranging from 'easy' to 'impossible'

1. Putting on socks or tights, without help or aids
2. Bending forward from the waist
3. Reaching up to a high shelf, without help or aids
4. Getting up out of an armless chair, unassisted
5. Getting up off floor from lying, without help
6. Standing unsupported for 10 minutes without discomfort
7. Climbing 12–15 steps without handrail or walking aid
8. Looking over shoulder without turning body
9. Doing physically demanding activities (e.g. gardening, sports)
10. Doing a full day's activities, at home or work

Source data from Calin et al, Bath Ankylosing Spondylitis Functional Index. Br J Rheumatol, Vol 34, 793–4 (1995).

The Dougados Functional Index (DFI) is an alternative validated instrument for the assessment of physical function in AS. The two instruments appear to have similar performance, with the BASFI quicker to administer than the DFI. Delayed diagnosis and increased disease duration are associated with higher BASFI scores, while lower BASFI scores have been shown to predict a better response to biologic therapies in axSpA patients. With conventional (non-biologic) treatment, the BASFI has been shown to increase by 0.5–1 units per year, so it is recommended that BASFI is checked every 3–6 months in clinical practice.

Spinal mobility

AxSpA can affect the spine at any level, so no single measure or movement can adequately assess the effect of structural damage and inflammation on spinal mobility. Combinations of measurements or composite scores are therefore required to assess spinal mobility in axSpA. Spinal mobility measures are clinician-assessed, and generally performed by physiotherapists outside of clinical trials.

The ASAS core set recommends the use of four separate measures to assess mobility at all spinal levels: occiput-to-wall distance (cervical mobility), chest expansion (thoracic spine), modified Schober test (lumbar forward flexion), and lateral lumbar flexion.

Bath Ankylosing Spondylitis Metrology Index

The Bath Ankylosing Spondylitis Metrology Index (BASMI) is an alternative and widely used measure to quantify the effect of axSpA on spinal mobility in an individual patient. This composite index includes measurements for the cervical spine (the tragus-to-wall distance and cervical rotation), lumbar spine (modified Schober test and lumbar side flexion), and hip mobility (intermalleolar distance), but not the thoracic spine (see Table 13.5 for a comparison between ASAS core set and BASMI). These individual measurements are then scored using either using pre-defined cut-offs on 3- or 11-point scales, or a linear function scale, to calculate a composite validated score ranging from 0 to 10. Higher BASMI scores indicate more severe limitation of movement.These investigations may only be practical in a specialist clinical setting with appropriately trained and resourced staff. The general recommendation is that spinal mobility or BASMI should be measured every 6–12 months. Spinal mobility measures and the BASMI have been shown to correlate well with radiographic damage. More details about the correct way to perform the spinal measures and calculate the composite BASMI score are available in the ASAS handbook on spondyloarthritis (Sieper, 2009).

Table 13.5 Comparison of mobility measures in ASAS core set and BASMI

Mobility being tested	ASAS core set	BASMI
Cervical spine	Cervical rotation	Cervical rotation
	Occiput to wall distance	–
	–	Tragus-to-wall distance
Thoracic spine	Chest expansion	–
Lumbar spine	Modified Schober test	Modified Schober test
	Lateral spine flexion	Lateral spine flexion
Hips	–	Intermalleolar distance

Peripheral joint assessment

The majority of patients with axSpA will have no peripheral joint involvement (see Chapter 7), so in clinical practice this assessment is not required in those patients with no peripheral joint involvement at their initial detailed examination and no subsequent symptoms. When peripheral joints are involved in axSpA, these frequently include the wrist, ankle, elbow, and sternoclavicular and metatarsal joints, which are not captured by the limited DAS28 score used in RA. The DAS28 is, therefore, deemed insufficient for assessment of peripheral joint involvement in axSpA, and a 44-joint count is recommended in axSpA. The presence of peri-articular involvement, in structures such as tendons, entheses and bursae, complicates peripheral joint counts and assessment in axSpA, as the joint count is only intended for involvement of the actual joint.

Enthesitis assessment

Enthesitis is an important component of axSpA, and spondyloarthritis (SpA) in general. Routine clinical assessments should include examination of the key entheseal sites for swelling and tenderness. However, correlation of clinical assessments with imaging is poor. A number of validated enthesitis scores exist in AS, including the Maastricht Ankylosing Spondylitis Enthesitis Score (MASES), the Berlin Enthesitis Index (also known as the Major Enthesitis Index), the Spondyloarthritis Research Consortium of Canada (SPARCC) and the Mander enthesitis indexes (Heuft-Dorenbosch, 2003). These scores are complex, involve the assessment of multiple sites and are relatively time-consuming, so are often not practical in busy clinics.

More recently, the Leeds Enthesitis Index has gained favor, particularly in the UK, as it is simpler and quicker to perform, involving only the presence or absence of enthesitis at the elbows (lateral epicondyles), knees (medial femoral condyles) and Achilles tendon insertions. This index was however developed and validated in psoriatic arthritis rather than axSpA. Enthesitis assessment is currently mainly performed in specialist SpA clinics and in clinical trials.

Quality of Life measures

The impact of axSpA on health-related quality of life can be measured using a number of instruments, although they are currently mainly used in clinical trials. The Ankylosing Spondylitis Quality of Life (ASQoL) tool is a self-reported questionnaire addressing the physical and psychological impact of the disease and includes items relating to sleep, mood, coping, relationships, social life, and activities of daily living. The original English ASQoL has subsequently been translated and validated in a number of other languages, as well as in patients with axSpA. More recently, the validated Evaluation of Ankylosing Spondylitis quality of life (EASi-QoL) has been proposed as an alternative measure, with superior responsiveness to treatment in routine clinical practice.

Fatigue measures

Fatigue is increasingly recognized as a key symptom in axSpA and reported as a major problem in two-thirds of patients, with a significant negative impact on quality of life, pain, and function (see Chapter 10). Therefore, fatigue warrants regular assessment and monitoring in clinical practice. A number of detailed fatigue questionnaires have been developed and used in clinical trials, but many of these are too unwieldy for use in routine clinical practice. Fatigue is already captured as part of the BASDAI, using a 100-mm VAS or 0–10 NRS, which provides a readily available measure for fatigue. A VAS score above 70 mm or NRS score above 7 is felt to represent significant fatigue.

Work productivity measures

There has been an increasing recognition that axSpA has a significant impact on a person's ability to work (covered in Chapter 10). Studies have demonstrated that effective therapy with TNF blockers has a positive effect on work productivity, so there is an increasing imperative to measure this in clinical practice, although this component was not included in the initial or revised ASAS core sets. It has become evident that simply measuring absenteeism from work is not sufficient as this significantly under-estimates the impact of axSpA on productivity while at work (presenteeism). Therefore, a number of instruments have been developed to measure the various aspects of the impact of axSpA on an individual's ability to work.

Work Productivity and Activity Impairment questionnaire in AS

The Work Productivity and Activity Impairment questionnaire in AS (WPAI:SpA) is a self-administered questionnaire developed to assess the impact of AS on productivity both at work and while doing daily activities over the previous week. The WPAI:SpA comprises six questions about employment status, hours of work missed due to AS or other reasons, hours actually worked, and the degree to which AS affected productivity at work and activities outside of work. The questionnaire generates scores for absenteeism (time off work), presenteeism (reduced productivity while at work), an overall work impairment score (combining presenteeism and absenteeism), and impairment of activities outside of work. However, these scores cover only a one-week period and are only valid in individuals who are employed.

Ankylosing Spondylitis Work Instability Scale

The Work Instability Scale for Rheumatoid Arthritis (WIS-RA; often also RA-WIS) was developed in an attempt to identify the 'at risk' period prior to work disability, where interventions might have greatest impact, in patients with RA. The WIS:RA was subsequently adapted and validated for AS (Ankylosing Spondylitis Work Instability Scale; AS-WIS) to identify those AS patients at risk of work disability or losing their job. The AS-WIS is a 20-item self-administered questionnaire with defined cut-offs for level of work instability. The predictive validity of AS-WIS for job retention is currently unknown.

Work Productivity Survey

The Work Productivity Survey (WPS) was developed to specifically assess the impact of arthritis on household and work productivity over a 1 month period. The WPS was recently also validated in axSpA following the initial validation in RA and psoriatic arthritis.

Work Limitations Questionnaire

The Work Limitations Questionnaire (WLS) is a more generic measure for assessing the impact of chronic health problems on work. The WLS captures limitations in a number of domains which include physical, mental, interpersonal, time management, and work output. The WLS allows for both an estimate of the amount of time the individual was limited while working, over the last 2 weeks, as well as an index which allows comparison of productivity compared to a 'healthy' employee.

While the current use of many of these instruments is largely restricted to clinical trials, the increasing recognition of the impact of axSpA on work productivity and the requirement for information to support the use of high cost therapies, suggest these may become more widely used in clinical practice in future.

Imaging to monitor axSpA

The use of imaging in the diagnosis of axSpA and AS is well established (covered in Chapters 11 and 12). The European League Against Rheumatism (EULAR) has published recommendations for the use of imaging in the diagnosis and management of axSpA (Mandl, 2015). Imaging also offers opportunities to monitor current disease activity (axial or peripheral), cumulative structural damage and complications in axSpA.

Imaging to monitor disease activity

MRI is the best widely available imaging modality to monitor axial disease activity. A number of studies have reported correlation of inflammatory changes on MRI with established clinical measures such as the BASDAI and ASDAS. However, there is currently insufficient evidence to recommend regular monitoring with MRI and no consensus on how frequently MRI scans should be performed to monitor the disease. In clinical practice, MRI scans (STIR sequences) of sacroiliac joints and the spine may be helpful to indicate whether or not a patient's current symptoms are likely to be due to active inflammatory disease. This may be particularly helpful where uncertainty exists when making decisions about starting or stopping biologic therapies for an individual patient. Nuclear bone scans should no longer be used to monitor disease activity in axSpA, due to the risks associated with these and the availability of safer alternatives such as MRI.

Where objective confirmation of disease activity in peripheral joints is required, MRI or ultrasound scans are generally the best modalities for this, with the choice largely dependent on local expertise and availability, and the anatomical site to be examined. It is likely that, in future, imaging may form part of treat-to-target strategies in axSpA.

Imaging to monitor structural damage and for musculoskeletal complications

ASAS and EULAR recommend that radiographs of the pelvis, and cervical, thoracic, and lumbar spine should be performed at the baseline clinic visit and may then be done on a regular basis to monitor progression of structural changes, but no more frequently than every 2 years. However, this is not routinely done in clinical practice due to concerns about radiation exposure associated with repeated x-rays. Many patients with axSpA will also never develop any significant structural or progressive radiographic changes. Certain circumstances clearly warrant spinal radiographs, such as the suspicion of a fracture following a fall, while pelvic x-rays are frequently used where hip disease is suspected in axSpA (see Chapter 7).

A number of spinal radiography scoring methods have been developed, including the Bath Ankylosing Spondylitis Radiology Index (BASRI) and modified Stoke Ankylosing Spondylitis Scoring System (mSASSS). However, these are intended for comparison between groups rather than monitoring changes in an individual, so their use is mostly restricted to clinical trials and cohort studies.

MRI is generally not a good modality for assessing structural bony changes, but may be helpful for detecting stress fractures or nerve root compression in patients with suggestive symptoms. While CT scans are excellent for assessing bony changes, they are only rarely used for this purpose in axSpA due to their significant radiation exposure. CT scans may be useful in detecting subtle spinal fractures where plain radiographs are normal following trauma (see Chapter 9 for more detail on spinal fractures in axSpA). CT scans have also been used in the past for guided sacroiliac joint steroid injections, but this has largely fallen out of favour since the introduction of TNF inhibitors.

Summary

AxSpA is a heterogeneous condition with multiple effects on patients. There are, therefore, a significant number of outcomes that could potentially be measured in patients with axSpA. Performing these in routine clinical practice has resource and logistic implications, so clinicians and teams looking after patients with axSpA need to decide which aspects they will monitor locally. ASAS has defined core data sets according to disease severity and treatments being used (Table 13.1). Most national and international guidelines for the use of biologics require regular monitoring of disease activity, so this has been widely incorporated into routine clinical practice in rheumatology secondary care services. Many of the outcomes used in axSpA are patient-reported, so these can be completed in advance of the clinic visit, while other measures may be done by physiotherapists. AxSpA is a slowly progressive condition, so longitudinal recording and review of outcomes is important to detect these changes and optimize management. As understanding of the natural history of the disease and imaging increases, it is likely that in future imaging will increasingly become incorporated into the long-term monitoring of axSpA. Regular monitoring will also be central in the inevitable move towards the stratified and treat-to-target approaches for axSpA in future.

Key References and further reading

Heuft-Dorenbosch L, Spoorenberg A, van Tubergen A, *et al.* Assessment of enthesitis in ankylosing spondylitis. *Ann Rheum Dis.* 2003;**62**(2):127–32. doi: 10.1136/ard.62.2.127.

Machado P, Landewe R, Lie E, *et al.* Ankylosing Spondylitis Disease Activity Score (ASDAS): defining cut-off values for disease activity states and improvement scores. *Ann Rheum Dis.* 2011;**70**(1):47–53. doi: 10.1136/ard.2010.138594.

Mandl P, Navarro-Compan V, Terslev L, *et al.* EULAR recommendations for the use of imaging in the diagnosis and management of spondyloarthritis in clinical practice. *Ann Rheum Dis* 2015;**74**(7):1327–39. doi: 10.1136/annrheumdis-2014-206971.

Martindale J, Shukla R, Goodacre J. The impact of ankylosing spondylitis/axial spondyloarthritis on work productivity. *Best Pract Res Clin Rheumatol* 2015;**29**(3):512–23. doi: 10.1016/j.berh.2015.04.002.

Sieper J, Rudwaleit M, Baraliakos X *et al.* The Assessment of SpondyloArthritis international Society (ASAS) handbook: a guide to assess spondyloarthritis. *Ann Rheum Dis.* 2009;**68**(Suppl II):ii1–44. doi:10.1136/ard.2008.104018

Zochling J. Measures of symptoms and disease status in ankylosing spondylitis. *Arthritis Care Res.* 2011;**63**(Suppl 11):S47–58. doi: 10.1002/acr.20575.

Chapter 14

Non-pharmacological treatment of axial spondyloarthritis

Key points

- While drugs play a key role in reducing disease activity, non-pharmacological therapies are crucial in maintaining function, flexibility, and quality of life. Therefore, non-pharmacological therapy remains a key component in the optimal management of axSpA, even in the era of biologics.
- Regular physical therapy allows patients to capitalize on the benefits of drug therapy and maintain optimal functional ability.
- Self-management and education strategies, supported by patient-support groups, facilitate independence, and quality of life in chronic diseases.
- A proportion of patients with severe disease may require hip or spinal surgery.
- It is hoped that the availability of more effective drug therapies will reduce the requirement for surgery in future.
- The optimal management of axSpa requires a combination of non-pharmacological and pharmacological treatments, for both initial and long-term management.

The main goals of treatment of axial spondyloarthritis (axSpA) are to reduce symptoms and maintain function. While drugs play a key role in reducing pain and stiffness associated with inflammation, as well as treating comorbidities, non-pharmacological therapies are crucial in maintaining function, flexibility, and quality of life. Non-pharmacological therapies are also required in order to maximize the outcomes and benefits associated with effective drug therapy. Therefore, the optimal management of axSpa requires a combination of non-pharmacological and pharmacological treatments, for both initial and long-term management.

Non-pharmacological therapy in axSpA can be broadly divided into:

- Exercise and physical therapy
- Self-management strategies and education
- Surgery

Exercise and physical therapy

Physiotherapy has always played a key role in the management of ankylosing spondylitis (AS) and prior to the development of TNF inhibitors, was the mainstay of therapy for chronic AS. The overall assumption is that regular exercise and stretching helps maintain function by preventing the development of ankylosis, although there is only limited evidence to support this assumption. These studies would require large numbers of participants and very long follow-up in order to detect significant differences.

Many of the physiotherapy interventions traditionally used in AS have a relatively limited evidence base. Studying complex interventions, such as physical therapy, in chronic diseases is complex, with difficulties relating to appropriate control groups, blinding, compliance, and outcomes. There are also limited commercial incentives for non-pharmacological interventions, compared to newer pharmacological therapies, so there are fewer and lower quality studies for these interventions. It should also be noted that most studies were performed prior to the Assessment in SpondyloArthritis international Society (ASAS) criteria for axSpA, so the available data relate mainly to patients with established AS.

A full review of various physiotherapy techniques used in AS is beyond the scope of this publication. The effect of physiotherapy in AS has been reviewed in a Cochrane systematic review which reported that physical therapy programmes are beneficial in terms of pain, function, spinal mobility, and patient global assessment (Dagfinrud, 2008). Supervised group physiotherapy (land or water-based) is better than individual home-based exercise, but both are better than no exercise intervention.

Various types of exercise (supervised group, home exercise, and global posture re-education) have been shown to be effective for pain, disease activity (BASDAI), function (BASFI), and mobility. Active exercise programmes are generally considered to be more beneficial than passive therapy, such as heat, ultrasound, and massage. There is evidence that balneotherapy (treatment by bathing) and spa therapies, particularly when combined with physiotherapy, are effective for pain, function, and disease activity in the short-term, but only limited data regarding the longer-term benefits or cost-effectiveness of this approach. With advances in technology, there is growing interest in alternative strategies to deliver individualized exercise programmes remotely using internet and app-based resources.

Self-management and education

Patient education and self-management are recommended as part of chronic disease management. In AS, patient education is considered to benefit pain and function, although there is only limited clinical trial data available to support this. Furthermore, education and behavioural therapy have beneficial effects on outcomes such as motivation and anxiety in AS and other chronic conditions, with some evidence to indicate this approach may also be cost-effective. There are no good studies on diet, probiotics, self-help groups, or lifestyle modification in AS, although these may play a role in the management of individual patients. In common with other musculoskeletal disorders, there is increasing interest in the use of mindfulness-based stress reduction and similar techniques, which have been shown to be beneficial for chronic pain, although these have yet to be evaluated in axSpA.

There are also a number of regional and national patient support and advisory groups, which many patients find helpful in terms of peer support and help in accessing appropriate healthcare services and disease-specific information. There is also an expanding community of people with axSpA on social media platforms, facilitating interactions with both other people with axSpA and healthcare professionals active in this domain.

Surgery

Surgery is generally considered as last-resort for AS and only required for a small minority of patients. It is anticipated, but not yet proven, that the availability of more effective therapies for axSpA will reduce the future requirement for surgery.

Surgery in AS typically involves the hips or spine. Some patients with AS have early and aggressive hip disease, so all patients should have their hips examined on initial presentation and when presenting with suggestive symptoms, although it can occasionally be difficult to distinguish hip pain from pain arising from the sacroiliac joints or spine (hip and peripheral joint involvement are covered in more detail in Chapter 7). Patients with disability or refractory pain and radiographic evidence of structural hip damage should be considered for total hip replacement, independent of age. Prospective cohort studies in AS report good pain relief and functional outcomes with hip surgery. Patients with AS who develop hip disease will often require hip replacements at younger ages than those with osteoarthritis, so choice of prostheses is influenced by considerations relating to durability and the possibility of future revisions. There is some evidence to suggest that the frequency of hip prosthesis surgery in Norway may be reducing since the introduction of TNF inhibitors for the treatment of AS (Nystad, 2014). Encouragingly, heterotropic bone formation and re-ankylosis after hip replacement are not increased in patients with AS, although preoperative non-steroidal anti-inflammatory drug prophylaxis is commonly used in AS.

Spinal surgery for AS should generally only be performed by surgeons or centres with expertise and experience of surgery in AS. Certain key principles of spinal surgery in AS differ from those in more common spinal surgery (Lazennec, 2015). Whenever spinal surgery is considered in AS, this should be carefully and individually evaluated by a specialist surgeon familiar with the potential benefits and associated risks, which need to be clearly communicated to the patient. Corrective spinal surgery in AS may be required for structural deformity leading to refractory symptoms or functional impairment that cannot be compensated, such as disabling kyphosis, loss of horizontal vision or painful spinal pseudoarthrosis. Surgery for correction of disabling functional deformity usually requires wedge osteotomy, which generally gives good functional outcomes, although complications and instrumentation failure are reported, particularly with polysegmental osteotomies. Instability due to spinal pseudoarthroses (also known as Andersson lesions) or spinal fractures generally require surgical fusion (spinal fractures are covered in more detail in Chapter 9). Far less commonly, spinal surgery is required for neurological complications such as spinal stenosis, myelopathy, or cauda equine syndrome.

Summary

Therefore, non-pharmacological therapy remains a key component in the optimal management of axSpA, even in the era of biologics. Regular physical therapy allows patients to capitalize on the benefits of drug therapy and maintain optimal functional ability. Self-management and education strategies, supported by patient-support groups, facilitate independence and quality of life in chronic diseases. While most patients will avoid the need for orthopaedic surgery related to their AS, a proportion of patients with severe disease may require hip or spinal surgery. It is hoped that the availability of more effective drug therapies to control disease activity in axSpA will reduce the requirement for surgery in future.

Key References and further reading

Dagfinrud H, Kvien TK, Hagen KB. Physiotherapy interventions for ankylosing spondylitis. *Cochrane Database Syst Rev.* 2008;(1):CD002822. doi: 10.1002/14651858.CD002822.pub3.

Lazennec JY, d'Astorg H, Rousseau MA. Cervical spine surgery in ankylosing spondylitis: Review and current concept. *Orthop Traumatol Surg Res.* 2015;**101**(4):507–513. doi: 10.1016/j.otsr.2015.02.005.

Nystad TW, Furnes O, Havelin LI, *et al.* Hip replacement surgery in patients with ankylosing spondylitis. *Ann Rheum Dis.* 2014;**73**(6):1194–7. doi: 10.1136/annrheumdis-2013-203963.

Chapter 15

Drug treatment for axial spondyloarthritis

Key points

- Pharmacological therapy for patients with axial spondyloarthritis (axSpA), especially those with severe disease, has been transformed by the introduction of the biologic therapies, and anti-TNF therapy in particular.
- Prior to 2005, treatment options for ankylosing spondylitis were limited to exercise therapy and non-steroidal anti-inflammatory drugs.
- The TNF inhibitors appear to have a good safety profile in axSpA, with no new safety signals.
- The high cost of innovator biologics remains an issue and it will be interesting to observe the effect of the introduction of multiple biosimilar TNF inhibitors in clinical practice.
- New therapeutics targeting different cytokine and signalling pathways should also become available over the next few years, so it remains to be seen what their role will be in the management of axSpA.

The pharmacological therapy for patients with axial spondyloarthritis (axSpA), especially those with severe disease, has been transformed by the introduction of the biologic therapies, and anti-TNF therapy in particular. Until approximately 2005, treatment options for ankylosing spondylitis (AS) were limited to exercise therapy and non-steroidal anti-inflammatory drugs (NSAIDs). Drug therapy prior to biologic therapies was largely focussed on treating symptoms and comorbidities such as uveitis and inflammatory bowel disease (IBD). The success of biologic therapies for rheumatoid arthritis (RA), and the subsequent demonstration of efficacy in both AS and non-radiographic axSpA (nr-axSpA), dramatically altered the outlook for patients with these chronic rheumatic conditions.

The requirement for, and choice of, drug therapy are largely determined by the severity and activity of the spondyloarthritis, the presence of associated comorbidities and the individual patient's preferences. While the treatment of patients with axSpA is generally coordinated by rheumatologists, effective management requires a multidisciplinary team approach with input from specialities outside rheumatology (such as gastroenterology, ophthalmology, and dermatology) (see Chapter 8 for more details on extra-articular manifestations).

Drug therapy for axSpA can be broadly classified into:

1. Analgesia and NSAIDs
2. Synthetic disease modifying anti-rheumatic drugs (sDMARDs)
3. Biologic therapy with anti-TNF agents

Analgesia and non-steroidal anti-inflammatory drugs

The main focus of treatment in axSpA is on controlling disease activity and maintaining function. While effective treatment often leads to a reduction in pain, many patients continue to have ongoing pain requiring additional treatment.

NSAIDs have a long history in AS and for many decades were the only proven drug treatment for axial disease in AS until the development of the biologic agents. Both traditional and cyclo-oxygenase-2 (COX-2) NSAIDs are effective for relieving pain, reducing stiffness, reducing disease activity (Bath Ankylosing Spondylitis Disease Activity; BASDAI), and improving function (Bath Ankylosing Spondylitis Functional Index; BASFI), with no significant differences in benefits or harms between NSAID classes reported in a Cochrane Systematic Review (Kroon, 2015).

Both COX-2 inhibitors and traditional NSAIDs are associated with increased gastrointestinal, renal, and cardiovascular events. A significant proportion of patients with axSpA will also have underlying IBD, which may also be a relative contra-indication to NSAID therapy in these patients due to concerns about aggravating IBD. However, this remains unclear and it is recommended to discuss the use of NSAIDs in these patients with their gastroenterologist (see also Chapter 8 for more details about IBD in axSpA). As always, the balance between potential benefit and harm with NSAIDs needs to be considered on an individual basis.

It should be noted that most guidelines for the treatment of AS and axSpA require patients to have had an inadequate response or intolerance to at least one, and usually a minimum of two, NSAIDS (unless contra-indicated) before being considered for biologic therapy. NSAIDs therefore remain first-line therapy for axSpA and are often the only drug therapy required for the majority of patients with mild-to-moderate disease.

There remains uncertainty regarding whether NSAIDs have a true disease modifying effect in AS. While a few studies suggested continuous or high-dose NSAIDs may be effective in slowing x-ray progression in patients with AS (Wanders, 2005; Poddubnyy, 2012), these were open-label or cohort studies. A recent randomized controlled trial (RCT) did not report any difference in radiographic progression of AS with continuous diclofenac compared to on-demand treatment (Sieper, 2015a).

Therefore, while NSAIDs had previously been recommended to be used regularly and at high doses, in the absence of convincing disease-modifying effect, it is difficult to support this strategy routinely for all patients, particularly in light of the known potential risks associated with long-term NSAID use and the availability of other effective therapies. For many patients, low dose or *pro re nata* (PRN; as necessary) use will be more appropriate.

There are no good studies of analgesics for the treatment of AS or axSpA. The general recommendation for musculoskeletal conditions is to use simple analgesics (such as paracetamol) and avoid opiate analgesics, where possible. Analgesics can generally be used on a PRN basis. It is also important to consider that there may be a number of potential causes for pain in people with axSpA, and all pain cannot automatically be assumed to be due to active disease. Existing damage or degenerative arthritis, particularly of the spine, may be difficult to distinguish from active axSpA and may require review by rheumatologists and possibly specialist imaging. A significant proportion of patients with chronic inflammatory arthritis may also have pain due to superimposed fibromyalgia, which may require additional specific treatment and interventions, as for primary fibromyalgia.

Corticosteroids

Systemic corticosteroids are generally not used or recommended for the treatment of axSpA. Corticosteroids are, however, used for some of the extra-spinal features and comorbidities of axSpA (see Chapter 8). Intra-articular injections may be used for rapid relief and treatment of peripheral arthritis, most typically knee effusions. Systemic or topical corticosteroids may also be used to treat flare-ups of uveitis or IBD, usually under the direction of ophthalmologists and gastroenterologists, respectively.

Synthetic disease modifying anti-rheumatic drugs

There is no good evidence to support the routine use of conventional sDMARDs (such as sulfasalazine or methotrexate) for the treatment of spinal symptoms or progression in axSpA (Chen 2013, 2014). Sulfasalazine has been used historically, but published data do not support efficacy for axial disease and its use is not recommended in treatment guidelines for axSpA. In one study which used sulfasalazine for the control arm in a TNF inhibitor study, up to 53% of patients who received sulfasalazine did achieve the primary end-point, but there was no placebo arm in this study (Braun, 2011).

However, in contrast to axial disease, sDMARDs may be effective for peripheral arthritis in patients with axSpA. Therefore, where biologic agents are readily available, sDMARDs are generally reserved for patients with peripheral arthritis, but may still be used more widely for axSpA in parts of the world where biologics are either unavailable or prohibited by costs (Benegas, 2012).

The most commonly used sDMARDs for peripheral arthritis in axSpA are sulfasalazine and methotrexate. Both of these drugs may also be effective for IBD and uveitis associated with axSpA. These drugs require regular safety monitoring blood tests (blood counts and liver function) and are associated with significant toxicity. Methotrexate is also teratogenic which limits its use in young women.

Biologic therapies

The development of biologic agents has revolutionized the treatment of inflammatory arthritis, including axSpA. The anti- TNF agents are currently the only licensed biologics for the treatment of both AS and nr-axSpA. With increased understanding of the pathophysiology of spondyloarthritis, new biologics targeting different pathways are likely to become available in the near future and are briefly mentioned here. In fact, at the time of writing, the IL-17 inhibitor, secukinumab, had just obtained its license for AS, heralding the start of this process. While the TNF inhibitors were initially adopted from RA, several other biologic agents used in RA have not proven efficacious in AS or axSpA.

Biologic agents are expensive and have specific safety screening and monitoring requirements, so are generally only prescribed by specialists with experience of these agents and conditions.

Anti-TNF agents

Pathophysiology studies had implicated a role for TNFα in AS and case reports suggested TNF blockers may be effective in AS, prompting larger phase III trials of a number of TNF inhibitors which were already in routine use for RA. The initial key RCTs were performed in patients who fulfiled the modified New York (mNY) criteria for AS (see Chapter 12). More recent studies have included patients meeting the broader Assessment of SpondyloArthritis international Society (ASAS) axSpA criteria. There are currently five innovator TNF inhibitors licensed by the European Medicines Agency (EMA) for AS and four for nr-axSpA with positive magnetic resonance imaging (MRI) and/or elevated C-reactive protein (CRP), although licensing varies slightly for other regulators. The TNF inhibitors currently licensed for AS and/or nr-axSpA are shown in Table 15.1.

The key phase III anti-TNF trials in AS and/or nr-axSpA are summarized in Table 15.2. Most anti-TNF studies required participants to have failed at least one NSAID prior to inclusion. The definition of 'active disease' required for eligibility in these trials varied, but was most commonly a BASDAI score and a spinal pain visual analogue scale ≥4 (see Chapter 13 for further information about these measures). As a result, most funders and national guidelines for the treatment of AS and axSpA require patients to have failed, due to inefficacy or intolerance, at least one NSAID (unless contraindicated) and have a BASDAI and spinal pain score of ≥4 prior to being considered for a TNF blocker. Furthermore, most treatment recommendations also require a predefined improvement in BASDAI, or other disease activity score, to be met for ongoing treatment with a particular anti-TNF agent. It should be noted that the primary endpoint in the phase III trials was typically the proportion of patients achieving an ASAS20 response, rather than improvement in BASDAI as used in clinical practice. This difference may be one of the factors contributing to the observation by many clinicians that response rates to TNF inhibitors in clinical practice are generally better than those reported in the phase III RCTs. An ASAS20 response is defined as an improvement of ≥20% and an absolute improvement of at least one unit, compared to baseline, in at least three of the following four domains, with no worsening in the remaining domain: physical function (measured using BASFI), spinal pain, patient global disease assessment, and inflammation (derived from questions 5 and 6 of BASDAI). The key ASAS response criteria are described in Table 15.3.

Infliximab (innovator tradename: Remicaide)

Infliximab is a chimeric (part mouse, part human) monoclonal antibody and was the first TNF inhibitor to demonstrate efficacy in patients with active AS. The ASSERT study reported that 61% of infliximab-treated patients with AS achieved an ASAS20 response at week 24 compared to 19% of placebo-treated patients (van der Heijde, 2005). Clinical benefit was observed with infliximab as early as week 2 and maintained with regular long-term therapy. Infliximab-treated patients also had improvement in physical function and quality of life, while adverse events were similar between the treatment groups. Infliximab is administered by intravenous infusion at 0, 2, and 6 weeks, then every 6–8 weeks. While in RA infliximab is typically used at a

Table 15.1 TNF inhibitors currently licensed for ankylosing spondylitis (AS) and non-radiographic axial spondyloarthritis (nr-axSpA). EMA = European Medicines Agency; MRI = magnetic resonance imaging; CRP = C-reactive protein

Generic name	Trade name	Administration route	Standard dose and frequency	Indication (EMA)
Innovator biologics				
Infliximab	Remicaide	Intravenous	5 mg/kg weeks 0, 2, 6, then 6–8 weekly	AS only
Adalimumab	Humira	Subcutaneous	40 mg every 2 weeks	AS and nr-axSpA (+ positive MRI and/or elevated CRP)
Etanercept	Enbrel	Subcutaneous	25 mg twice weekly *or* 50 mg once weekly	AS and nr-axSpA (+ positive MRI and/or elevated CRP)
Certolizumab	Cimzia	Subcutaneous	400 mg weeks 0, 2, 4 then 200 mg fortnightly	AS and nr-axSpA (+ positive MRI and/or elevated CRP)
Golimumab	Simponi	Subcutaneous	50 mg monthly (100 mg monthly for weight >100kg)	AS and nr-axSpA (+ positive MRI and/or elevated CRP)
Biosimilars				
Infliximab biosimilar	Inflectra or Remsima	Intravenous	5 mg/kg weeks 0, 2, 6, then 6–8 weekly	Same as for infliximab innovator: AS
Etanercept biosimilar	Benepali	Subcutaneous	50 mg once weekly	Same as for etanercept innovator: AS and nr-axSpA (+ positive MRI and/or elevated CRP)

Table 15.2 Seminal phase III trials of TNF inhibitors for ankylosing spondylitis (AS) and non-radiographic axial spondyloarthritis (nr-axSpA)

Active drug	Study population	Study name	Sample size	Primary outcome	Primary result (active vs placebo)	Duration (weeks)	Reference
Infliximab	AS	ASSERT	297	ASAS20	61.2% vs 19.2%	24	van der Heijde (2005)
Adalimumab	AS	ATLAS	315	ASAS20	58.2% vs 20.6%	12	van der Heijde (2006a)
Adalimumab	nr-axSpA (included AS on review)	ABILITY1	185	ASAS40	36% vs 15%	12	Sieper (2013)
Etanercept	AS	–	356	ASAS20	ETA 50mg 1x/week 74.2%; ETA 25mg 2x/week 71.3% vs placebo 37.3%	12	van der Heijde (2006b)
Etanercept	AS (note: control = sulfasalazine, no placebo)	–	566	ASAS20	ETA 75.9% vs sulfasalazine 52.9%	16	Braun (2011)
Etanercept	Early nr-axSpA (<5 years; central scoring)	EMBARK	215	ASAS40	32.4% vs 15.7%	12	Dougados (2014)
Certolizumab	AxSpA (nr-axSpA and AS) *plus* elevated CRP and/or positive MRI	RAPID-AxSpA	325	ASAS20	57.7% (200mg Q2W); 63.6% (400mg Q4W) vs 38.3%	12	Landewe (2014)
Golimumab	AS	GO-RAISE	356	ASAS20	59.4% (50mg); 60.0% (100mg) vs 21.8%	14	Inman (2008)
Golimumab	nr-axSpA (central scoring)	GO-AHEAD	197	ASAS20	71.1% vs 40.0%	16	Sieper (2015b)

Table 15.3 Assessment in Ankylosing Spondylitis (ASAS) 20% and 40%response criteria

Response criteria (abbreviation)	**Description**
ASAS improvement criteria	Based on change in the following 4 domains: ◆ Physical function (measured by BASFI; Box 13.1) ◆ Spinal pain (VAS/NRS) ◆ Patient global assessment (Table 13.4) ◆ Inflammation (derived from questions 5 and 6 of the BASDAI relating to morning stiffness; see Table 13.2)
ASAS 20% response criteria (ASAS20)	◆ Improvement of ≥20% and at least one unit, compared to baseline, in at least 3 of the 4 domains *and* ◆ no worsening in the remaining domain.
ASAS 40% response criteria (ASAS40)	◆ Improvement of ≥40% *and* at least two units, compared to baseline, in at least 3 of the 4 domains *and* ◆ no worsening in the remaining domain.

dose of 3 mg/kg every 8 weeks (after the loading dose), the licensed dose for AS is 5 mg/kg every 6 weeks. This has cost implications compared to other TNF inhibitors and has resulted in some national guideline bodies not recommending innovator infliximab (tradename Remicaide) for the treatment of AS. This is likely to change with the introduction of infliximab biosimilars (discussed elsewhere) which will be priced lower than Remicaide and the other innovator TNF inhibitors.

Adalimumab (innovator tradename: Humira)

Adalimumab is a fully humanized anti-TNF monoclonal antibody and is administered subcutaneously at 40 mg every 2 weeks. The ATLAS study reported that 58% of adalimumab-treated patients with active AS achieved an ASAS20 response at 12 weeks compared to 21% of those who received placebo (van der Heijde, 2006a). The ABILITY-1 study sought to evaluate the efficacy and safety of adalimumab in patients with only nr-axSpA by using the ASAS criteria for axSpA (covered in more detail in Chapter 12) and then excluding patients with existing x-ray changes fulfiling mNY criteria for AS (Sieper, 2013). Overall 36% of adalimumab-treated patients achieved the primary outcome ASAS40 response (≥40% improvement in ASAS response criteria) at week 12 compared to 15% who received placebo. However, when x-rays were re-read centrally, a significant proportion (~35%) were in fact identified as having radiographic changes consistent with AS, rather than nr-axSpA. Subsequent reanalysis of the results suggested that the treatment benefit was mainly driven by benefit in the patients with AS rather than in nr-axSpA patients. These factors account in part for the initial divergent license approvals for adalimumab for the treatment nr-axSpA by the EMA (positive) and the US Food and Drug Administration (FDA) (negative). It has subsequently also been recognized that patients with nr-axSpA are more likely to respond to a TNF inhibitor if they have a positive MRI and/or elevated CRP (i.e. objective evidence of inflammation). The total sample size of 185 included 43 patients who had nr-axSpA but neither a positive MRI nor an elevated CRP.

Etanercept (innovator tradename: Enbrel)

Etanercept is a soluble fusion protein containing the extracellular domains of two TNF receptors which bind and neutralize TNF. Several large phase III studies confirmed the efficacy of subcutaneous etanercept for the treatment of AS. Etanercept 50 mg once weekly was shown to be as effective as etanercept 25 mg twice weekly, with ASAS20 response rates of 74% and 71%, respectively, compared to 37% in those who received placebo (van der Heijde, 2006b). A separate study demonstrated that etanercept (50 mg once weekly) was significantly more effective for the treatment of AS than sulfasalazine, with ASAS20 response rates of 76% with etanercept compared to 53% with sulfasalazine (Braun, 2011). A number of subsequent studies have confirmed sustained clinical efficacy and improvement in function and health-related quality of life with etanercept treatment, while one study has reported that etanercept was associated with clinically relevant NSAID-sparing effects.

The EMBARK study evaluated the efficacy of etanercept in patients with early nr-axSpA who fulfilled the ASAS criteria for axSpA but not the mNY radiographic criteria and who had symptom duration <5 years (Dougados, 2014). The ASAS40 response rate at 12 weeks was 32% for the etanercept-treated patients compared to 16% for the placebo group. Post-hoc analysis suggested higher etanercept response rates in patients with higher baseline CRP levels and/or confirmed sacroiliitis on MRI.

Certolizumab (innovator tradename: Cimzia)

Certolizumab is a PEGylated humanized antigen-binding fragment of an antibody and is administered subcutaneously. The RAPID-axSpA study investigated the efficacy of two dosing regimens of certolizumab and was the first RCT to examine the efficacy of an anti-TNF agent across the spectrum of patients with active axSpA, including patients with both AS and nr-axSpA (Landewe, 2014). Patients had to fulfil the ASAS criteria for axSpA and, in addition to a BASDAI score ≥4, they also had to have an elevated CRP and/or sacroiliitis on MRI. The ASAS20 response rate was achieved at 12 weeks by 58% (200 mg every 2 weeks) and 64% (400 mg every 4 weeks) of participants who received certolizumab compared to 38% who received placebo. Improvements with certolizumab were similar in the AS and nr-axSpA subpopulations, with improvements observed as early as 1 week in this study. Certolizumab also led to sustained improvements in function, work productivity, and quality of life, with no significant differences in adverse events between groups.

Golimumab (innovator tradename: Simponi)

Golimumab is a fully human monoclonal antibody administered by subcutaneous injection. The GO-RAISE study reported that 59–60% of the patients with AS treated with golimumab 50 mg or 100 mg every 4 weeks achieved an ASAS20 response at week 14 compared to 22% of patients who received placebo (Inman, 2008). The subsequent GO-AHEAD study evaluated the efficacy of golimumab in nr-axSpA by recruiting patients who fulfiled the ASAS criteria for axSpA and then excluding those who had radiographic changes (using central scoring) fulfilling mNY criteria for AS (Sieper, 2015b). Overall 71% of patients treated with golimumab 50 mg achieved an ASAS20 response at 16 weeks compared to 40% of placebo-treated patients. The differences in response were greatest in patients with objective signs of inflammation defined as a positive MRI or elevated CRP, while there was no significant difference in patients with negative MRI and normal CRP. Golimumab, like etanercept, adalimumab and certolizumab is therefore licensed by the EMA for nr-axSpA in patients with positive MRI and/or elevated CRP. The golimumab responses in patients with AS were sustained long-term, with no new safety signals.

Biosimilar TNF inhibitors

Biosimilars (also known as 'follow on biologics' or 'subsequent entry biologics') are biologic products that are required, by most regulatory authorities, to demonstrate proof of similarity of effect to the licensed innovator product, but not *de novo* efficacy. Biosimilars are also subject to indication extrapolation, meaning that the biosimilar licence applies to all the same indications as the innovator reference biologic, without requiring dedicated RCTs for each indication.

The comparable efficacy of the infliximab biosimilar, CT-P13 (tradenames: Inflectra, Remsima), with innovator infliximab was demonstrated for RA in the PLANETRA study (Yoo, 2013), and due to indication extrapolation is therefore not required to be repeated for AS. The PLANETAS study demonstrated pharmacokinetic equivalence at steady state of CT-P13 and innovator infliximab in patients with AS, with no statistically significant differences in the secondary ASAS20 response rates at week 14 or 30 (week 14 ASAS20 63% for CT-P13 and 71% for innovator infliximab) (Park, 2016). An indirect meta-analysis reported similar efficacy of the infliximab biosimilar compared to the other TNF inhibitors.

An etanercept biosimilar (tradename: Benepali) has recently also been licensed and become available in the UK and EU. This biosimilar demonstrated equivalence with innovator etanercept in RA, with a comparable safety profile (Emery, 2015). As the pharmacokinetics of etanercept are comparable in RA and AS, the EMA extrapoloated the authorization for Benepali to the approved therapeutic indications for Enbrel, which include AS and nr-axSpA (in patients with positive MRI and/or elevated CRP).

Many other biosimilar versions of innovator TNF inhibitors are currently undergoing evaluation and likely to reach the market over the next few years. The exact role and positioning of biosimilars in the treatment of axSpA in clinical practice remains to be seen and will ultimately be influenced by cost, demonstration of sustained efficacy and long-term safety.

Choice of TNF blocker

In the absence of head to head trials, the choice of anti-TNF agent for a particular patient with axSpA is largely based on comorbidities, cost, and patient preference. Specifically, the soluble receptor protein etanercept is not effective in IBD, unlike the monoclonal antibody TNF inhibitors. In the absence of any differentiating efficacy or safety signal, drug cost is likely to become the main determining factor when choosing an anti-TNF agent to use in axSpA, or any of the other rheumatic conditions, particularly with the arrival of cheaper biosimilar TNF inhibitors (covered elsewhere in this chapter).

Switching and stopping TNF inhibitors

Not all patients will respond to a particular TNF inhibitor. While switching to an alternative anti-TNF agent is recommended in cases of intolerance (provided this is not due to a class effect), the situation is less clear for inefficacy to the first agent. There are no RCTs to inform this decision, but there is now increasing data from registries and observational studies to support the use of sequential TNF blockers for axSpA, which is now generally included as an acceptable treatment option in updates of treatment recommendations for axSpA. As with other rheumatic conditions, the response rate with each subsequent TNF blocker reduces, but still appears worth pursuing in carefully selected patients where other causes of apparent 'inefficacy' (such as fibromyalgia) have been excluded. The response rate to first TNF blocker appears to be considerably higher in clinical practice than the rates reported in the phase III clinical trials, so in clinical practice switching is a relatively infrequent requirement.

While TNF inhibitors should generally be switched or stopped in those patients with no clinical response by 6 months of treatment, withdrawal of TNF inhibitors in patients in apparent remission is not recommended. Several studies have shown that the majority of patients will relapse within 1 year of discontinuation, with most flaring up within the first 4–10 weeks of discontinuation. Intermittent or 'on-demand' dosing has been shown to only marginally reduce costs, at the expense of worse clinical outcomes, so is also not recommended. However, there is increasing interest in reducing the dose or frequency of TNF inhibitors in patients in remission, with several studies evaluating this approach in RA and axSpA.

Radiographic progression with TNF inhibitors

While TNF inhibitors unequivocally slow radiographic progression in RA, the initial phase III open-label extension studies in AS did not report any reduction in radiographic progression with treatment up to two years with TNF inhibitors, when compared with progression in historical AS controls. In fact, there were even suggestions that syndesmophyte formation may be increased in the short-term. These findings led to a number of mechanistic hypotheses, including a potential uncoupling of inflammation and new bone formation (see Chapter 5). However, more recent observational studies and longer follow-up of study participants, have suggested that TNF inhibitors may indeed slow radiographic progression, particularly in earlier disease (Zhang, 2015).These different results are likely to relate to differences in trial design, the definition of radiographic progression (erosions or new bone formation), and the longer treatment and observation period required for the slow evolution of radiographic changes in AS (compared to the more rapid changes seen in RA).

Other biologics currently used for RA

It should be noted that the apart from TNF inhibitors, the other biologic agents currently used in routine clinical practice for the treatment of severe RA are not licensed for AS or axSpA. Rituximab (anti-CD20 monoclonal antibody) and abatacept (co-stimulation inhibitor) demonstrated no convincing evidence of efficacy in a small nationwide study and open-label pilot study, respectively. Interestingly, phase II-III studies of two anti-IL-6 receptor monoclonal antibodies (tocilizumab and sarilumab) somewhat surprisingly failed to reach their primary end-points (ASAS20) or demonstrate efficacy in AS, despite a significant reduction in CRP levels. The role of IL-6 inhibition in SpA is currently being re-evaluated in new studies.

New and future biologic therapies

With advances in the understanding of the pathogenesis and genetic associations of AS and related conditions, several new biologic and small molecule inhibitors are currently undergoing evaluation and will be available in the clinic in the near future.

IL-12/23 and IL-17 inhibitors

There has been particular interest in the IL-17/IL-23 (Th17) axis which has been increasingly implicated across the spondyloarthritis spectrum (see Chapters 4 and 5). Several approved agents targeting this pathway are already established in clinical practice for the treatment of psoriasis and psoriatic arthritis.

Secukinumab

Secukinumab is a highly selective, fully human monoclonal antibody targeting the pro-inflammatory cytokine IL-17A. The efficacy of subcutaneous secukinumab in patients with active AS was demonstrated in the linked phase III MEASURE studies (Baeten, 2015). MEASURE 1 used an intravenous secukinumab loading regimen and reported ASAS20 response rates at week 16 of 60–61% for the two subcutaneous secukinumab doses (75 mg and 150 mg) compared with 29% for placebo. MEASURE 2 used a subcutaneous secukinumab loading regimen and reported ASAS20 response rates at week 16 of 41% for secukinumab 75 mg, 61% for secukinumab 150 mg and 28% with placebo, with significant improvements sustained through 52 weeks. These studies led to the approval of subcutaneous secukinumab 150 mg by the EMA (November 2015) and FDA (January 2016) for the treatment of active AS. It should be noted that this dose is lower than the licensed dose (300 mg) typically used in the treatment of psoriasis. There were no significant new safety signals in the phase III trials, but the long-term safety and role of secukinumab remains to be determined, particularly in patients with associated IBD.

Several other anti-IL-17 agents are also in development for AS and a range of other inflammatory conditions.

Ustekinumab

Ustekinumab is a subcutaneous monoclonal antibody targeting the p40 subunit of both IL-12 and IL-23. Ustekinumab is licensed for the treatment of psoriasis and psoriatic arthritis. An open-label, single-arm trial suggested potential efficacy of ustekinumab in active AS, although the results of phase III RCTs are still awaited at the time of writing.

Agents specifically targeting IL-23, but not IL-12, directly or via the p19 subunit are also in development.

New small molecule inhibitors and oral agents

Apremilast

Apremilast is an oral phosphodiesterase 4 inhibitor licensed for the treatment of active psoriasis and psoriatic arthritis. While a small phase II study of apremilast in AS failed to reach its primary outcome (change in BASDAI at week 12), the secondary clinical and biomarker results suggested it may be effective in AS and further studies were undertaken. The results of the recently completed phase III study are awaited.

Janus kinase (JAK) inhibitors

Many pro-inflammatory cytokines bind to cytokine receptors resulting in signal transduction via the janus kinase (JAK) family of enzymes and STAT transcription factors. Drugs that inhibit the activity of JAKs therefore have the potential to block cytokine signalling. A number of small molecule JAK inhibitors are currently undergoing trials for a range of rheumatic conditions, although their efficacy and safety in AS remains to be determined.

Summary

There have been major advances in the treatment of AS and, more recently, nr-axSpA. In particular, the TNF inhibitors have transformed outcomes for patients with this condition. While there was initially some uncertainty regarding the ability of these agents to delay radiographic progression in AS, it now seems increasingly likely that this will be the case. It is hoped, but remains to be seen, if TNF inhibitors will do the same in nr-axSpA, thereby effectively preventing patients from developing the radiographic changes that define AS. It should, however, be noted that a significant number of patients with nr-axSpA will never progress to AS, regardless of treatment (see Chapter 3). These agents appear to have a good safety profile in axSpA, with no new safety signals. The high cost of innovator biologics remains an issue and it will be interesting to observe the effect of the introduction of multiple biosimilar TNF inhibitors in clinical practice. New therapeutics targeting different cytokine and signalling pathways should also become available over the next few years, so it remains to be seen what their role will be in the management of axSpA. There will, therefore, be multiple options available for the treatment of patients with axSpA and one of the major challenges going forward will be to determine how best to use these agents in clinical practice, with hopes for better stratification in future.

Key References and further reading

Baeten D, Sieper J, Braun J *et al.* Secukinumab, an Interleukin-17A inhibitor, in ankylosing spondylitis. *N Engl J Med* 2015;**373**(26):2534–48. doi: 10.1056/NEJMoa1505066.

Benegas M, Muñoz-Gomariz E, Font P, *et al.* Comparison of the clinical expression of patients with ankylosing spondylitis from Europe and Latin America. *J Rheumatol* 2012;**39**(12):2315–20. doi: 10.3899/jrheum.110687.

Braun J, van der Horst-Bruinsma IE, *et al.* Clinical efficacy and safety of etanercept versus sulfasalazine in patients with ankylosing spondylitis: a randomized, double-blind trial. *Arthritis Rheum* 2011;**63**(6):1543–51. doi: 10.1002/art.30223.

Chen J, Veras MM, Liu C, *et al.* Methotrexate for ankylosing spondylitis. *Cochrane Database Syst Rev.* 2013;**28**;2:CD004524. doi: 10.1002/14651858.CD004524.pub4.

Chen J, Lin S, Liu C. Sulfasalazine for ankylosing spondylitis. *Cochrane Database Syst Rev.* 2014;**11**:CD004800. doi: 10.1002/14651858.CD004800.pub3.

Dougados M, van der Heijde, Sieper J, *et al.* Symptomatic efficacy of etanercept and its effects on objective signs of inflammation in early nonradiographic axial spondyloarthritis: a multicenter, randomized, double-blind, placebo-controlled trial. *Arthritis Rheumatol.* 2014:**66**(8):2091–102. doi: 10.1002/art.38721.

Emery P, Vencovský J, Sylwestrzak A, *et al.* A phase III randomised, double-blind, parallel-group study comparing SB4 with etanercept reference product in patients with active rheumatoid arthritis despite methotrexate therapy. *Ann Rheum Dis.* 2015 Jul 6 doi: 10.1136/annrheumdis-2015-207588. [Epub ahead of print].

Inman RD, Davis JC, vad der Heijde D, *et al.* Efficacy and safety of golimumab in patients with ankylosing spondylitis: results of a randomized, double-blind, placebo-controlled, phase III trial. *Arthritis Rheum.* 2008;**58**(11):3402–12. doi: 10.1002/art.23969.

Kroon FP, van der Burg LR, Ramiro S, *et al.* Non-steroidal anti-inflammatory drugs (NSAIDs) for axial spondyloarthritis (ankylosing spondylitis and non-radiographic axial spondyloarthritis). *Cochrane Database Syst Rev.* 2015;7:CD010952. doi: 10.1002/14651858.CD010952.pub2.

Landewe R, Braun J, Deodhar A, *et al.* Efficacy of certolizumab pegol on signs and symptoms of axial spondyloarthritis including ankylosing spondylitis: 24-week results of a double-blind randomised placebo-controlled Phase 3 study. *Ann Rheum Dis.* 2014;**73**(1):39–47. doi: 10.1136/annrheumdis-2013-204231.

Park W, Yoo DH, Jaworski J, *et al.* Comparable long-term efficacy, as assessed by patient-reported outcomes, safety and pharmacokinetics, of CT-P13 and reference infliximab in patients with ankylosing spondylitis: 54-week results from the randomized, parallel-group PLANETAS study. *Arthritis Res Ther.* 2016;**18**(1):25. doi: 10.1186/s13075-016-0930-4.

Poddubnyy D, Rudawaleit M, Haibel H, *et al.* Effect of non-steroidal anti-inflammatory drugs on radiographic spinal progression in patients with axial spondyloarthritis: results from the German Spondyloarthritis Inception Cohort. *Ann Rheum Dis* 2012;**71**:1616–22. doi: 10.1136/annrheumdis-2011-201252.

Sieper J, van der Heijde D, Dougados M, *et al.* Efficacy and safety of adalimumab in patients with non-radiographic axial spondyloarthritis: results of a randomised placebo-controlled trial (ABILITY-1). *Ann Rheum Dis* 2013;**72**(6):815–22. doi: 10.1136/annrheumdis-2012-201766.

Sieper J, Listing J, Poddubnyy D, *et al.* Effect of continuous versus on-demand treatment of ankylosing spondylitis with diclofenac over 2 years on radiographic progression of the spine: results from a randomised multicentre trial (ENRADAS). *Ann Rheum Dis.* 2015a pii: annrheumdis-2015-207897. doi: 10.1136/annrheumdis-2015-207897. [Epub ahead of print].

Sieper J, van der Heijde D, Dougados M, *et al.* A randomized, double-blind, placebo-controlled, sixteen-week study of subcutaneous golimumab in patients with active nonradiographic axial spondyloarthritis. *Arthritis Rheumatol.* 2015b;**67**(10):2702–12. doi: 10.1002/art.39257.

van der Heijde D, Dijkmans B, Geusens P, *et al.* Efficacy and safety of infliximab in patients with ankylosing spondylitis: results of a randomized, placebo-controlled trial (ASSERT). *Arthritis Rheum.* 2005;**52**(2):582–91. doi: 10.1002/art.20852

van der Heijde D, Kivitz A, Schiff MH, *et al.* Efficacy and safety of adalimumab in patients with ankylosing spondylitis: results of a multicenter, randomized, double-blind, placebo-controlled trial. *Arthritis Rheum.* 2006a;**54**(7):2136–46. doi: 10.1002/art.21913.

van der Heijde D, Da Silva JC, Dougados M, *et al.* Etanercept 50 mg once weekly is as effective as 25 mg twice weekly in patients with ankylosing spondylitis. *Ann Rheum Dis.* 2006b;**65**(12):1572–7. doi: 10.1136/ard.2006.056747.

Wanders A, van der Heijde D, *et al.* Nonsteroidal antiinflammatory drugs reduce radiographic progression in patients with ankylosing spondylitis: a randomized clinical trial. *Arthritis Rheum.2005*;**52**(6):1756–65. doi: 10.1002/art.21054.

Yoo DH, Hrycaj P, Miranda P, *et al.* A randomised, double-blind, parallel-group study to demonstrate equivalence in efficacy and safety of CT-P13 compared with innovator infliximab when coadministered with methotrexate in patients with active rheumatoid arthritis: the PLANETRA study. *Ann Rheum Dis.* 2013;**72**(10):1613–20. doi: 10.1136/annrheumdis-2012-203090.

Zhang JR, Liu XJ, Xu WD, *et al.* Effects of tumor necrosis factor-α inhibitors on new bone formation in ankylosing spondylitis. *Joint Bone Spine.* 2015 pii: S1297-319X(15)00261-4. doi: 10.1016/j.jbspin.2015.06.013. [Epub ahead of print].

Chapter 16

The current and future outlook for patients with axial spondyloarthritis

Key points

- There have been major advances in axial spondyloarthritis (axSpA) over the past decade. The current and future outlook for patients with axSpA is therefore much improved and largely positive.
- There is still significant unmet need in pathophysiology, prevention, diagnosis, and treatment.
- While several new therapeutic agents are expected to reach the clinic over the next few years, the treatment of individual patients is likely to remain largely empiric for the foreseeable future.
- There is a need for the development of biomarkers and stratified treatment approaches in order to capitalize on previous gains for the benefit of our patients.

There have been significant advances in axial spondyloarthritis (axSpA), particularly over the past decade. As such, both the current and future outlook for patients with axSpA is much improved and largely positive. There is however still significant unmet need in axSpA.

Pathogenetics

The genetic and immune mechanisms that underlie axSpA are starting to unravel. It is likely that further progress will not only identify new therapeutic targets, but also yield information that is of prognostic and diagnostic value. In addition to new pharmaceutical interventions, a better understanding of the complex interactions with the microbiome and biomechanics will likely also facilitate the development of novel lifestyle and dietary interventions for axSpA. While a cure for axSpA, or any of the chronic rheumatic conditions, seems unlikely in the foreseeable future, we may be moving closer to being able to reliably identify those at high risk of developing the disease, thereby facilitating the development of potential interventions that attempt to prevent disease development.

Diagnosis

As outlined in other chapters, particularly Chapter 12, there remains significant unmet need in diagnosis. Despite the advances in imaging and classification criteria, there continues to be a significant delay from symptom onset to obtaining a diagnosis of axSpA, so further work is required to educate the public and those healthcare professionals who come into contact with these patients early in the course of their condition. It is likely that advances in imaging technology and better understanding of the natural history of the imaging changes in axSpA will help address some of these issues. Accurate and timely diagnosis has significant implications due to the availability of effective, but expensive therapies for axSpA. It also remains to be seen if earlier diagnosis and, therefore, earlier treatment will lead to genuine long-term benefits in axSpA.

Treatment options

The TNF inhibitors have transformed the treatment of axSpA and are generally well tolerated. However, use of these agents is limited by cost, so it will be interesting to observe the effect of the cheaper, but still expensive, biosimilar agents reaching the open market. Furthermore, it is still unclear whether there will be significant treatment or safety differences between the biosimilar drugs and their innovator versions in real-world practice. Further work is also required to establish the optimal long-term maintenance dose of biologic drugs in axSpA, particularly for those with low disease activity or in remission.

Several new therapeutic agents for axSpA are already undergoing phase II and III trials, with more to follow. There will therefore be a very welcome range of alternative treatment options available for patients with axSpA in the near future. However, it is unclear how best, and in what order, to use these agents in clinical practice. There are currently no reliable biomarkers of response to inform choice of treatment, so this should be a research priority. Due to the nature of the disease, it is also possible that optimal biomarkers for axSpA may involve advances in molecular imaging, rather than soluble laboratory biomarkers as may be the case for other rheumatic conditions. The early phase studies suggest that the next wave of therapeutic agents for axSpA will have similar, but not significantly better, responses than the current TNF inhibitors. This is somewhat disappointing as the current level of primary outcome responses in axSpA clinical trials are relatively modest (i.e. ASAS 20% or 40% responses), particularly compared to some of the high hurdle responses that are being reported in conditions like psoriasis with the IL-17 inhibitors (i.e. 90–100% responses), so there is clearly a need for more effective drugs, rather than just more drug options.

Treatment strategies

The treatment of rheumatoid arthritis (RA) has been transformed not only by the development of biologic agents, but also by the use of aggressive treat-to-target strategies, particularly in early disease. While a similar approach has been advocated for axSpA, there is, to date, very limited evidence to support this strategy. Specifically, the natural history of axSpA is less predictable and more heterogeneous than that in RA, so aggressive treatment strategies risk unnecessarily 'over treating' a significant number of patients. A treat-to-target strategy also requires an achievable, validated target to aim for and proof that aggressive treatment is truly disease modifying, which still remain to be fully established for axSpA. While imaging targets (i.e. treating until no inflammation is evident on imaging) are superficially appealing for axSpA, these require a detailed understanding of the natural history and implications of imaging changes to avoid unnecessarily treating normal imaging variants or biomechanical responses. Ultimately, it is likely that a more subtle stratified or precision medicine approach will be required for axSpA, rather than a simple treat-to-target approach.

In summary, while significant advances have been made on every level in axSpA, there remains a need for further advances in order to capitalize on these gains and optimize the outcomes for those people with, and those at risk of, this condition in future.

Index

page numbers in bold refer to figures and tables